COMPASSIONATE CARE: NAVIGATING DEMENTIA TOGETHER

HOW TO BE CONFIDENT AND INFORMED IN THE CARE OF YOUR LOVED ONE, ACCESS TOOLS TO PROVIDE THE BEST QUALITY OF LIFE, MAINTAIN YOUR WORK-LIFE BALANCE

L E SUMMERS

CONTENTS

COPYRIGHT

DEDICATION

To my dearest mother,

This book is a tribute to your unwavering strength and the love that flowed through you. As I delve through the depths of dementia, I am reminded of our journey together—the highs and lows, the moments of confusion and clarity, and the unbreakable bond we shared.

You faced the relentless grip of dementia with courage and grace, teaching me the true meaning of resilience. Through your unwavering spirit, you taught me the power of embracing each day, no matter how challenging it became. Your unwavering love and determination inspired me to embark on this journey of understanding, to shed light on the complexities of dementia.

In this book, I strive to honor your memory and the countless others who have faced this formidable foe. I hope that by sharing our story, I can offer solace, guidance, and a glimmer of hope to those who are navigating this path.

Mom, your legacy lives on in every word of this book. You may have been taken from us by dementia's grip, but your spirit endures in my heart. Through this book, I hope to raise awareness to help bring a world where no one faces dementia alone.

This dedication is a testament to the extraordinary woman you were— a beacon of love, strength, and resilience. Thank you for the indelible mark you left on my life, and may your light continue to shine brightly, illuminating the path for others who face the challenges of dementia.

I will always love you, Mom.

INTRODUCTION

Being a caregiver is an act of love. You are offering your time, patience, skills, and often your own happiness to be there for someone else. In an ideal world, you'd be able to attend courses about dementia and talk to professionals about the best course of action. Not everyone can afford that, though. Caregiving isn't an exact science; you should focus on learning from your mistakes and from those who did this before you.

Caregivers have to deal with several issues: Knowing someone you love is changing, and the dread of not knowing enough about dementia and how to handle each challenge. Of all caregivers who care for senior loved ones, 48% have to deal with dementia or Alzheimer's Disease. Even with insurance, 70% of the lifetime costs of dementia fall on family members (*ADI - Women as Carers: Gender Considerations and Stigma in Dementia Care*, n.d.).

This can be an exhausting journey, and it will make you question things you used to take for granted. Family feuds arise during this period, but you need to consider what's better for the person needing care. They need to fulfill their activities of daily living and can't wait until the entire family comes together.

Don't feel guilty if you're not always capable of giving 100%. But knowing what lies ahead is the first and most important step toward making the best of the situation.

Whether you have a small or a big family, it's nice to have people who you can count on during difficult situations. That could be financial help, someone you can talk to about your issues or someone who you can call to take care of the dementia patient when you are stuck in traffic. You will also find people who refuse to donate their time or their assistance, claiming they already have enough problems. These are usually the first ones who step forward to dispute any decision you make on your own.

I wrote this book to connect with people who feel overwhelmed, alone, and lost in their new role as a caregiver. Sometimes, coping with a loved one with dementia may feel like too much. I've been there, and understand the pressure to be taking care of someone, offering emotional and psychological support, while also managing your personal life. Bad feelings may arise at these moments, and if you let them take control, they will make everything even more difficult.

You will need to learn and adapt as quickly as possible. Things are going to change fast, and you have to adapt just as fast. I'm here to tell you it's possible to go through that entire process without giving up on self-care.

In this book, you will learn the most important steps for those who need to care for a loved one with dementia. The first stage is dealing with diagnosis, then learning the many stages of the disease. You will have to manage the work of nurses and other professionals, and other members of the family who agree to help. As you navigate through the different stages, you will gain practical knowledge that applies to the person you're caring for.

Among all caregivers in America today, 70% are women who start out at the age of 49 (*ADI - Women as Carers: Gender Considerations and Stigma in Dementia Care*, n.d.). Dementia is more common among Hispanic and African-American seniors. People with different cultural backgrounds deal with dementia in their own way, which can affect care and family agreements. Depending on the previous relationship between the caregivers, that could become even more complicated.

A dementia diagnosis impacts family relationships, possibly leading to feuds and even legal disputes. Caregivers have their own life to balance, and their relationships with their children and spouses could suffer from that new arrangement, not to mention their professional lives. It's difficult to meet deadlines and be diligent in your job.

The work situation can also turn sour because caregivers take a lot more responsibility into their lives when parents have dementia. Medical costs are also a problem, whether or not the parent has insurance. Family caregivers struggle to balance work and the new responsibilities, falling behind with deadlines, missing opportunities, and becoming less productive at work.

I'm here to tell you that you are not alone and that it's possible to stay sane and happy while caring for a loved one with dementia. This book is my effort to share what I learned and provide much needed support to others who handle a dementia patient. As a 68-year-old family caregiver who spent over three years looking after my late mom when she had dementia, I have made many mistakes and learned from them.

Beginning about six years earlier, my father had gradually taken over the care of my mother as she started her progression, then with the help of a lovely nurse who visited them twice a day, doing those things that he could not. With his demise, I came to be my mother's caregiver in 2019. That required me to travel across the country to my childhood home from many years ago. After three years as a caregiver, I learned what I'm going to share with you. It was more challenging than I imagined, but my mother appreciated my help, which made it worth it. Seeing my mother express her gratitude with words or just a glimmer in her eye when she saw me each day meant the world to me.

With limited support, I took on the task of caring for my bed-ridden mom, who had once been a renaissance woman, well-versed in keeping a home, who was a fantastic artist/crafter, active in the community, and who raised two outstanding children. It wasn't easy to see her mind regress the way it did, but I embraced the challenge, learned everything I could about this disease, and offered my mother the treatment she deserved.

That's the knowledge that I now plan to share with you. I will offer practical alternatives to handle every moment, helping you to understand the disease and its effects on you and your loved one. You'll also find the nine steps you need to be the primary caregiver for your loved one with dementia. With the tools I'll give you, you can develop a supportive environment that will help you to see the silver lining in all of this.

Time to start our journey!

DEALING WITH THE DIAGNOSIS
THAT CHANGES EVERYTHING

*T*he first time you hear that diagnosis, it's hard not to be scared. You'll know that things are going to change, and you shouldn't expect yourself or your loved one to react kindly to hearing the news. That diagnosis doesn't come at once; it may take months of tests and exams to get there. Try to remain optimistic during that period, but also be aware of possible outcomes.

Only 40% of individuals discuss dementia symptoms before they show (*What Is Alzheimer's*, n.d.). Meanwhile, 70% of elderly individuals would love an early diagnosis if it can improve the quality of their lives (*Alzheimer's Disease Facts and Figures*, n.d.).

Talk frankly about this matter with your loved ones, and start building your support base well in advance of the diagnosis. It's important to know who will be there for you and how you can contact them in difficult times.

WHAT IS DEMENTIA?

Dementia is a type of condition that affects the cognitive functions of the brain to the point that it hinders people from living their daily lives normally. It's not one disease, such as Alzheimer's, but a term that serves to organize a series of conditions that lead to similar changes in behavior. Just as the word *fracture* could be applied to several bones in your body, dementia can also apply to different diseases.

Dementia affects the ability of remembering, reasoning, and thinking and also changes a person's personality traits. A person in the most advanced stages of dementia is incapable of living by themselves and needs help to nourish, dress, clean, and perform other basic activities by themselves.

The cause of dementia is not always apparent, which can make the treatment difficult. Studies haven't yet shown what factors can prevent dementia, though some health issues—such as tumors, high blood pressure, and vitamin deficiencies—can make it worse. Still, it's important to detect dementia in its early stages and to begin treatment as soon as possible. That will help you plan for the future and to give the best possible assistance to your loved one.

Dementia manifests itself when the nerve cells in a person's brain cannot connect with each other normally causing the brain cells to die at an abnormal rate. While 60–80% of dementia cases are caused by Alzheimer's (World Health Organization: WHO, 2023), they are not the same thing. Dementia is an umbrella term that consists of several diseases, including vascular dementia, dementia with Lewy Bodies, and diseases that cause degeneration of the frontal lobe of the brain (frontotemporal dementia). Other causes of dementia include autoimmune diseases, alcohol abuse, strokes, physical brain injuries, and nutritional issues.

Dementia is more common in people 65 years or older, but that doesn't make it a natural part of aging. Many people reach much older ages without developing dementia, and there have been cases of dementia in young people. Some factors increase the chances of developing dementia, such as hypertension, diabetes, obesity, drinking, smoking, depression, and a sedentary lifestyle. As the brain cells continue to die, it becomes harder for the person to process thoughts and do simple chores. Dementia may not affect consciousness, but it has an impact on a person's mood, behavior, and emotional control.

It's important to watch your loved one and notice any signs that could mean they're in the early stages of dementia. They may show signs of confusion and disorientation, even in familiar places, getting stuck making simple decisions or solving simple problems.

If any of those issues arise, take them to a doctor, who will examine vital signs such as blood pressure and ask for a battery of laboratory tests. These tests will show if there's any imbalance in the patient's system that could lead to dementia. It's also important to keep detailed records of one's medical history. A history of dementia in the family can predispose your loved one to develop it themselves.

Alzheimer's

Alzheimer's is a progressive disease, and it becomes worse without proper treatment—which is why it's so dangerous to think of it as a normal part of life. It starts with mild loss of cognitive abilities, but in its later stages, the person can lose touch with the world around them. Alzheimer's patients tend to live for four to eight years after diagnosis but can reach even 20 years (*What Is Alzheimer's?*, n.d.).

By attacking the part of the brain related to learning, Alzheimer's affects short-term memory, causing confusion and disorientation. The person with Alzheimer's has a hard time noticing there's something wrong with their mind. They may become suspicious of those around them, stop recognizing people they have known their entire lives, and in extreme cases, have difficulty speaking, swallowing, and walking.

Vascular Dementia

This kind of dementia happens when there's damage to the blood vessels that carry oxygen to the brain, affecting cognition and brain function. There are cases of vascular dementia coming on gradually and also of sudden attacks that continue to progress gradually. Vascular dementia's symptoms are close to Alzheimer's, and it can happen at the same time as other types of dementia.

It's possible to identify the brain abnormalities that cause vascular dementia through MRI scans. It is common in people who have already suffered strokes. Cerebrovascular diseases are often related to cardiovascular disease, though research on the matter is still inconclusive.

Lewy Body Dementia

Lewy body dementia (LBD) is one of the most common causes of dementia, affecting people of age 50 or older, though it can happen in younger people. LBD is hard to diagnose since its symptoms are confounded with other brain diseases. The fact that LBD often happens along with other brain disorders complicates the diagnosis even more.

It is caused by a protein called alpha-synuclein which, in abnormal quantities, can deposit in the brain and affect its chemical balance. It impacts mood, behavior, movement, and thinking. At first, LBD is mild, with the patient being able to take care of themselves, and it grows to a stage in which they depend on others for assistance and care.

Scientists are still trying to find a cause for LBD. They know that it's associated with the loss of neurons that produce neurotransmitters—the connections between brain cells. The most common risk factor is age, but Parkinson's disease and REM sleep behavior disorder also influence this type of dementia.

Frontotemporal Dementia

Also called frontotemporal disorders, or FTD, this kind of dementia happens when neurons in the frontal and temporal lobes of the brain are damaged. It happens in people between their 30s and 60s, making it difficult to speak and to have social interactions. FTD patients get agitated and engage in repetitive and obsessive behaviors.

Mixed Dementia

The term mixed dementia is used for people who have two or more different diseases that cause dementia symptoms. One in every ten dementia patients suffer from more than one type (*What Is Mixed Dementia?*, n.d.), most commonly Alzheimer's disease and vascular problems. One of these types will be predominant, which can be identified by its symptoms being more acute than the other ones.

LATE dementia

Scientists have only recently characterized Limbic-predominant Age-related TDP-43 Encephalopathy (LATE) as a form of dementia. It's caused by a brain cluster of TDP-43 protein, a substance that also causes other types of brain disorders. LATE attacks people of over 80, and it can only be diagnosed after death with an autopsy.

Other Diseases That Affect Dementia

Dementia can also result from other diseases, trauma, or risk factors that have a direct or indirect impact on the brain. The risk factors include age, family history, Down syndrome, and low levels of certain nutrients. A simple fever caused by an infection and immune disorder can damage brain cells. Side effects of certain medicines can also cause dementia-like symptoms.

Some of the diseases that can cause dementia include:

- Huntington's disease: A disease that affects the nervous system, causing neurons to deteriorate. Patients are usually between their 30s and 40s.
- Traumatic brain injury (TBI): A condition common in soldiers and athletes, caused by repetitive hits in the head. Depending on the part of the brain that's injured, it could cause dementia or a series of different psychiatric symptoms.
- Creutzfeldt-Jakob disease: A rare and fatal disease caused by prions, infectious proteins that deposit in the brain. It affects people after age 60 and can be passed down from parents.
- Parkinson's disease: People who have had Parkinson's for over a year can develop dementia symptoms.

DEMENTIA SYMPTOMS

Dementia results from many causes, diseases, and risk factors. It's challenging to pinpoint which cause your loved one has.

More important than that is getting them diagnosed early enough if they haven't been already. Dementia is a progressive disease, and the sooner you detect it, the more you can do for the person who's suffering from it.

Most dementia symptoms have to do with memory, communication, reasoning, attention, judgment, and problem-solving. Watch out for these signs:

- Having trouble solving problems and completing tasks.
- Having difficulty with words, whether expressing themselves through speaking and writing, or understanding others by listening and reading.
- Mixing up old memories.
- Repeating the same question over and over.
- Calling familiar objects and people by the wrong name.
- Having trouble tracking time.
- Having trouble with balance and movement.
- Showing a lack of interest in their activities.
- Losing consideration for other people's feelings.
- Being confused by familiar situations.
- Having hallucinations, delusions, and paranoia.
- Being unable to make decisions.
- Forgetting recent events.
- Spending more time than usual to fulfill simple tasks.
- Being irresponsible with money.
- Getting lost walking or driving on a familiar route.
- Being impulsive.
- Losing or misplacing objects.

NORMAL AGING VERSUS DEMENTIA

For a long time—and even to this day—people have treated Alzheimer's as a common factor of aging. They look at the behavioral changes in an old person as senility and even find it amusing. In reality, despite aging being one of the most important factors in Alzheimer's, the disease isn't inherent to old age, and can even affect younger people.

People acquire certain behaviors as they age, but the intensity of those behaviors is indicative of dementia. Since the most common reason for dementia in people over 65 is Alzheimer's, we can make a parallel between the two. For example, people who are aging normally can make strange decisions once in a while, lose track of time, and forget something only to remember it later. For a person with Alzheimer's that behavior becomes recurrent. They make poor decisions all the time, have difficulties remembering the time of the day or the year, and forget important things permanently.

When that kind of behavior becomes apparent, you need to take your loved one to the doctor. The first thing they're going to ask is for a physical checkup. Cognitive and neurological tests can be conducted at a psychiatrist's office. They comprise problems of varying levels of difficulty that challenge the patient's mental skills, including memory, problem solving, reflexes, balance, sensory response, and their language and mathematical skills. A psychiatric evaluation also serves to detect changes in behavior and mood, and to diagnose depression, which is one of the principal causes of dementia.

You may want to consult your family's doctor or a psychiatrist when your loved one's behavior starts to change, but the diagnosis should be made by a neurologist or a psychiatrist who specializes in geriatric patients. Ask for references from other doctors and people who have been through the same situation.

Specialists aren't cheap, and they are not as easy to find as they should be. If you can't find or afford one, contact the neurology department of a medical school. You can also look for help at the National Institute of Aging (NIA), which provides support for aging research.

The first step of the diagnosis is to rule out any other condition that might mess with the patient's cognitive functions. These conditions may or may not be treatable, and it's important to get them out of the way. Doctors also interview the patient and their families about how and when the symptoms arose and check their medical history to see if there's any injuries, diseases, or medication that may be affecting their brain. Doctors also ask if there are any cases of dementia in the family, which can be a determining factor.

Tests that need to be applied at a laboratory include computed tomographies and brain scans, which can detect any anomaly inside the brain tissues, such as tumors or strokes. Brain scans can produce images of the brain through fields and radio waves (magnetic resonance imaging) or radiation (positron emission tomography). Blood tests by themselves are not the most efficient way of diagnosing dementia but can assist other types of tests. A blood test can show a high level of beta-amyloid, a protein that's common in people with Alzheimer's. These tests are not covered by insurance, and they can be costly.

Getting an early diagnosis will allow you to plan for the treatment and legalities with the participation of your loved one, if they're still capable of that. It also gives you time to prepare yourself, to get used to the idea of being a caregiver, and to get practical information about the challenges that lay ahead.

A complete diagnosis should not only confirm that your loved one has dementia but what kind of dementia they have. This is valuable information for caregivers and care workers, who can then provide the specific type of care and support that the patient needs. The differences between these different types may be subtle for a layperson, but they will affect the treatment.

The dementia patient can also benefit from an early diagnosis, allowing them to continue their independent life as long as possible. They can also build their relationship with professional caregivers and nurses and strengthen their bond with family members. With an early diagnosis, a patient can start saving money for the future, deal with their legal matters, and start with their drug and non-drug treatments, which are more efficient in the early stages of dementia.

Getting a dementia diagnosis for yourself or a loved one is still a scary scenario. The disease affects the social lives and careers of everyone involved. It's important to be firm and realistic when facing this news, and think of the diagnosis of a positive development. Knowing the problem is the first step to solving it.

It's important that your loved one is informed about their condition, even if they're afraid of it. Here are five arguments you can present to receive the news of a dementia diagnosis:

1. An informed patient has a say in the decisions regarding their own health, and they can have a more active participation while they're still in the early stages of dementia.
2. Dementia treatments are more effective during the early stages, which include not only medication but many alternative therapies that require the patient's active participation.
3. An early diagnosis gives you time to make important legal and financial decisions without being questioned.
4. You can stand your ground and show that having dementia doesn't mean you're useless, and you can use that to raise awareness about this condition.
5. You can get in contact with other people with dementia, share your experiences with them, and help to fight prejudices.

As a caregiver, it's also your job to fight this sort of prejudice. People with dementia are often mistreated and kept away from society. There are no universal human rights standards created specifically for people with dementia, but they're still human beings and deserve dignity.

HOW TO MEASURE DEMENTIA

Each dementia case is different and happens at its own pace. Still, several models have classified the different stages of dementia. The most basic one is divided into three phases—mild, moderate, and severe—which describe the early, middle, and final stages of the disease.

This model doesn't comprise all the nuances of dementia, and other more detailed models have been created. These are the Functional Assessment Staging Test, the Clinical Dementia Rating, and the Global Deterioration Scale for Assessment of Primary Degenerative Dementia (DementiaCareCentral.com, 2023).

Functional Assessment Staging Test (FAST)

Dementia is a journey, and it's difficult to tell the stages of any journey while you're going through it. The Functional Assessment Staging Test (FAST) is based on the patient's ability to conduct their daily activities. These seven stages aren't written into stone, but they offer a road map of what lies ahead. You may find that your loved one is stuck for years in a stage, or that they skipped another one, but that's natural. Use this as a guide, adapting it to your own necessities.

Normal Behavior

People with Stage 1 of dementia show no symptoms of memory loss and function normally, although their brains might still be changing. They can stay in this stage for years until the first symptoms appear.

Forgetfulness

People start to forget the names of people and things and to misplace objects around the house, being unable to remember where they put them. The memory loss is still mild, and the family may mistake it for normal memory deterioration related to old age.

Mild Decline

It's during this stage that families begin to realize that there's something wrong going on. Forgetfulness becomes a serious problem, the patient has a hard time concentrating; they get lost in their own neighborhood, and have a hard time finding words. Mild decline can go on for up to seven years, and it's important to look for help as soon as possible.

Moderate Decline

By this point, most families have already figured out that these symptoms aren't just normal aging. The dementia patient can no longer manage their finances or remember recent events. They know there's something wrong with them, entering a state of denial about their symptoms. This stage can last up to two years, and most patients get their diagnosis here.

Moderately Severe Decline

At this point, the dementia patient needs assistance with some of their daily chores, such as dressing or bathing. They might have a hard time remembering their own address and phone number, or what time of the year it is. Still, they have a vivid image from things that happened a long time ago, such as their childhood. They will repeat themselves during conversations, and will ask the same question several times. In these moments it's important not to lose patience, and repeat the answers as many times as necessary. Moderately severe decline can last around 18 months, during which memory deficiencies are a serious issue.

Severe Decline

Patients at this stage need constant supervision at their residence. They won't be able to perform activities of daily living (ADL) on their own, and will need help to bathe and dress. Recent and past events escape their memory, and they also have trouble remembering the names of their loved ones. They also have trouble controlling their bladder, have trouble speaking and often have anxiety and delusions. It's still possible to connect with them, as long as you have patience and treat them with love and respect. You can reach them by reading a fairy tale from a book, for example. Even if they can't understand the story, they can appreciate the cadence of your voice. This stage can last for up to two years.

Very Severe Decline

This is the final stage of dementia, and most people pass away before they reach it. Here, patients need help 24/7 with all their activities, such as feeding and hygiene. They also lose their capacity to speak and communicate, as well as their motor skills, and the ability to walk.

Clinical Dementia Rating (CDR)

CDR evaluates the patient through a five-point system that's based on their cognitive abilities in the following areas:

- memory
- orientation
- judgment and problem-solving
- community affairs
- home and hobbies
- personal care

The results of this exam are used globally through a standardized score. Since the test involves long interviews with the patient and their families, results take some time, but they are still considered valuable by health professionals around the world.

Global Deterioration Scale

The Global Deterioration Scale (or Reisberg Scale) divides cognitive decline into seven stages (DementiaCareCentral.com, 2023). It better serves patients with Alzheimer's or other types of dementia that includes memory loss. After interviewing the patient and their family, the doctor evaluates which stage they're in. Patients in stages 1-3 are not diagnosed with dementia, stage 4 is classified as early dementia, stages 5 and 6 middle dementia, and stage 7 classified as late dementia.

CHAPTER 1 PRACTICAL EXERCISE

These are dementia diary prompts for one week that will help you discover whether your loved ones show signs and symptoms.

Sunday

- Can your loved one remember what they had for breakfast?
- When people come to visit, does your loved one remember their name?

Monday

- When your loved one needs to go to the bathroom, can they find it by themselves?
- Have they been repeating the same questions?
- Do they insist they're not in their own house?

Tuesday

- Do simple decisions elude your loved one?
- Can they track their time?
- Has your loved one been unusually rude?

Wednesday

- Is your loved one taking decisions by impulse?
- Do you notice them losing their balance?
- Are they having trouble completing simple tasks?

Thursday

- When your loved one talks about their past, do they blend different stories?
- Are they losing interest in things that once caught their attention?
- Are they misplacing objects?

Friday

- Are your loved ones having trouble expressing themselves?
- Do they make exaggerated gestures while trying to find the right words?
- Are they neglecting their personal hygiene?

Saturday

- Is your loved one experiencing paranoia?
- Are they uncomfortable in familiar situations?

Depending on the results of this test, you might want to take your loved one to a medical professional to evaluate if they have dementia, and which state they are in.

 Caregiving often calls us to lean into love we didn't know was possible.

— TIA WALKER

Caring for your older parent or patient will already help you overcome many of the mental challenges you're facing once you hear about dementia. You'll love yourself for standing by them in this journey and be proud of what you have accomplished.

However, the second step requires another challenging time: taking care of necessary responsibilities first.

There will always be doubts and questions. You will think of things you should have done before, things you should have done better, and things you should have avoided from the beginning. Those voices are always in our minds, no matter what we do—it's part of being human!

You are already doing something great. Don't torture yourself if you're not doing it perfectly. This isn't a mathematical problem that you can solve if you know the right steps. Each case of dementia offers its challenges, and you have to figure out the way as you go. The best way of doing it is by being kind to yourself—always!

2

HANDLING THE CHALLENGING
RESPONSIBILITIES AND
LEGALITIES FIRST

here's no time to lose. You can start to take care of the legal matters regarding your loved one's disease before their definitive diagnosis. Legal matters are like little monsters that grow up without you seeing them, and if you don't watch out, they are going to bite you hard later on. Find a lawyer who you trust, if possible, one who specializes in elder law, and discuss your situation.

Don't waste time. As soon as you get the diagnosis, start to take care of some important matters. It's time to be strong, to put aside your emotions, at least for the moment, and do what must be done. Some of these decisions will be hard, and they will put your mental health to the test. There will always be those who will question your actions having nothing to offer.

The advice I'll give you here doesn't substitute for the services of a licensed attorney. Estate planning attorneys have the competency to answer all of your questions, and if you don't have a referral to one, you can contact your local bar association. It's important to do this while your loved one has as many faculties available to them as possible. That means it's ok to put this book down and come back once you've had one or more meetings with an attorney.

Locate and secure all necessary legal documents—such as wills, trusts, contracts, etc.,—that your loved one has entered for the past five years. This will allow the attorney to check their legal validity and effectiveness, including before this time period that affects your loved one's property and legal rights. Getting copies of health, life, and long-term care insurance policies is also important, including details about their current value and the names of the owners, account holders, and beneficiaries. Keep your family informed of any legal conversations, for it might have an impact on the disposition of their own estate.

FAMILY TIES

People with dementia need love and affection as much as any other person would, though their way of expressing those feelings might change. They often express their affection awkwardly at the wrong time and in the wrong place. That can be an issue and embarrass other people, especially if they don't know the person is sick.

Dementia may erase memories from a person's mind, but it doesn't delete their past. People may still have a grudge against the patient, and they might have reasons not to like them. Not everyone can put that aside as they watch the mind of the dementia patient fade away. Some may hide their animosity because they are interested in getting compensation after the person dies.

Caregivers may find that their role in the relationship has changed in many ways. They are now in charge of finances, legal matters, house maintenance, meal preparation, and other responsibilities that used to fall on their loved one's shoulders.

Families might not be happy with this change of roles and could accuse you of trying to take advantage of that situation.

Be prepared for a change in your social life as well. You won't get as many visits from friends as before. Not everyone is ready to carry on a conversation with a dementia patient. It takes patience and a good deal of affection to answer the same question several times in a row without losing your temper. You won't be able to hang out with your friends as much as you did before. You can arrange with a relative to take care of the dementia patient the night you're invited to go out, however, this is an even bigger responsibility than taking care of a child.

Not everyone is ready to fulfill caregiver tasks, but dementia won't wait until people are prepared. Sons and daughters are often expected to fulfill their needs, but they are not always available, having families to take care of and issues of their own. The responsibility may also fall on the shoulders of the husband or wife, which can be a problem because of their own age and health problems.

Your family still needs to function and be happy. While the dementia patient becomes the center of all of your efforts, you can't neglect your spouse, siblings, and most of all, the children in your family. They need as much attention as before, and if you don't make an effort to be there for them, it will have an impact on their lives.

Even little children can notice when their relative has dementia, and that might frighten them. It's important to tell them that dementia is not contagious and that there's no reason to be embarrassed if their parents or grandparents with dementia don't always remember who they are. Counselors and social workers can help with that.

It's easy to judge people who are not helping, but you should remember that every person has their own obstacles in life, and that can get in the way of caregiving. Talk to them without accusations, and explain that if they can't be there to bathe or clothe the dementia patient, they can at least show up for a cup of coffee once or twice a week—that makes a huge difference!

For some people, the more they do for the dementia patient, the guiltier they feel for not being able to do more. That guilt can come from many places, such as not having a good relationship with that person throughout their lives, not having taken seriously the symptoms of dementia as they arose, or the feeling of abandoning them if they have to commit them to a hospital or residential care.

As the caregiver, your opinions should prevail in family decisions since you are in the front row. Still, you don't want your family members to feel you're imposing your own ideas without hearing them. A good idea is to have regular meetings in which you can explain what's going on, and everyone can then offer ideas and solutions to the family's problems.

Feuds may already exist before the diagnosis. You must know how to handle these issues when they arise. With an early diagnosis, loved ones with dementia can participate in the decision-making while they're still in the middle stages of the disease. It's better to have these decisions on record so that later, when members of the family start to question each other's decisions, they can prove that this is the will of their loved one.

In any situation in which two or more people can't agree about money issues, it's wise to get third-party help from a financial adviser. Communication problems may arise, and it's important that everyone has their say and is able to talk to each other without interference. Face-to-face or phone conversations are better in that regard than exchanging texts through apps or email.

When it comes to dementia itself, each person may try to present their own ideas and solutions. Not everyone will agree with the diagnosis, and someone might want to consult their own specialists. Others will argue that their loved one is just going through the normal stages of aging, while others will go to the other extreme and start to make plans for the funeral, even if the person is still in the early stages.

As the primary caregiver, you need to be firm and practical. Ask the doctor for a detailed written report, and if necessary, take your relatives to the doctor's office to get all the information they need. You need the sympathy of these people, for they're the ones who are going to be by your side when things get ugly.

Imagine you pay a professional to take care of your loved one while you're at work. The professional leaves at the time you arrive home. One day, you get stuck in traffic, and the caregiver can't stay much longer. You need assistance from one of your relatives to fill that gap. The closest person is your nephew, with whom you had a fight over inheritance. Will you be able to call them and ask them to take care of that person?

Having a dementia diagnosis can be like exploding dynamite at the bottom of a swamp; you never know what's coming to the surface. People will fight for money, control, and even childhood issues may arise. You can't lose focus on what matters the most, which is the physical and mental well-being of the person who has dementia.

Someone has to be the bigger person, and it might as well be you. Try to bring everyone together around the same mission, which is giving your loved one the care that they need to navigate this terrible disease. It may take some persuasion and a few awkward family conferences, but you need to make it work.

Not every family can afford in-home care. The government may offer some assistance, but that's not always enough. It's important that the family talk about money matters when it comes to giving your loved one the best possible care. Someone might have to postpone a trip, cancel their tennis lessons, or sell something valuable. What's crucial is that these sacrifices don't come all from one person but are done by all family members equally.

Bringing a neutral third party to this situation could be a suitable solution. Get someone who isn't a part of the family and who isn't biased toward any of the family members. They will iron out issues regarding the family's finances and the medical expenses for the loved one with dementia.

There are often those who think that the entire issue is overblown, that this is just a way for you to get attention from your parents, and that they don't need all that care. If they need to hear about it from the doctor, make an appointment for them to hear it from the professional's mouth.

With an early diagnosis, the dementia patient can express their wishes in writing, whether they accept being committed to a hospice at the late stages of dementia or if they want to be at home under the care of a relative. This document will prevent more arguing between the family members about what they're supposed to do.

An only child will have to take most of the responsibility of caregiving on their own, but there are caregivers with plenty of siblings who still have to do most of the caring by themselves. That doesn't happen only because the siblings are selfish, but it can happen because of a lack of communication. If people don't know you're going through difficulties, they can't help you.

Some family members can't donate their time and be there in person, but they can contribute to make things easier. That could be sending money for groceries and other bills, offering accounting services, doing research to find the best doctors and treatments, offering supplies such as geriatric diapers and equipment such as wheelchairs—the list goes on.

At times it may be difficult to treat your family members with respect, especially in those days in which you are about to lose hope. Nobody asks to be in this situation, and each person reacts in their own way. You may not agree with all opinions, and you may feel that they aren't giving as much as you are. You can disagree with each other regarding the stages of the disease and financial decisions. Keep in mind that you don't have all the answers, and try to avoid burning bridges.

Think of these family conferences as business meetings rather than family get-togethers. You are there to bring attention to and discuss a problem. A good idea might be to prepare some slides, if you are computer savvy, to show the evolution of your loved one's condition, the next steps in the treatment, and how much time, money, and effort you'll need for it. Hear other people's questions and let them comment before explaining how each one can help in the situation.

Communication shouldn't stop at the end of the meeting. An online app group is great for keeping in contact with all the family members in real-time. It allows you to share information and to ask for help. Many families already have a group like that, but it's best to have one only dedicated to news and requests related to the dementia patient.

Since the caregiver is the closest person to the dementia patient, other members of the family may accuse them of manipulating their loved one to get more from an inheritance. Nothing makes a family fight more than an aging parent who needs care, and the dementia patient will be the biggest victim of that fight.

Caregiver burnout is a serious issue that can arise when a person has to take care of a loved one's personal needs while also judging the egos and judgments of the family. That makes it hard to maintain a positive approach to something that's already difficult and leads to physical, emotional, and mental exhaustion. There's also the problem of the lack of money since most families can't afford all the medical needs of a loved one, and the government doesn't offer much assistance in that regard.

For many caregivers, spending time and money on themselves comes with a dose of guilt. They see themselves as guardians of their loved one, and the family might also pressure them in that regard. When families meet to discuss the needs of the dementia patient, they should also talk about the needs of the primary caregiver and what kind of support they're willing to provide for them. Paying for a caregiver's therapy may be as important as buying packs of diapers for the dementia patient.

DEALING WITH LEGALITIES

In law, the term legal capacity refers to the ability to make rational decisions and to understand the consequences. As dementia progresses, the patient is robbed of their legal capacity, but in its early stages, they are still able to carry out, sign, and execute a document. A doctor's report can prove whether the person still has their legal capacity to validate documents such as a will.

A lawyer should then explain the meaning and consequences of that document to the dementia patient. While it's possible to sign some legal documents without the presence of a lawyer, having one will prevent the document from being contested in the future. You might already have a family lawyer, but it's best to have a specialist in elder law who will help you navigate through the nuances of the process.

Suspicions might arise when you step up to the responsibilities of caring for your loved one with dementia, which complicates family relationships. For example, the responsible caregiver has to help their loved one prepare all the legal documents—the legal documents that the dementia patient signs while in the first stages of the disease allow others to make decisions for them when they can't do it anymore.

A lawyer with experience in geriatric law is the best person to determine if legal capacity is required to validate a signature, which can vary between different legal documents. Sometimes you might need a doctor's evaluation to determine the level of legal capacity. You need to discuss the document with your loved one, making sure that they understand its contents and the consequences of signing them.

You should assess any documents that were completed and signed in the past and review them to see if they need updating. Some legal documents can be completed without a lawyer, but even then, it helps to get legal advice, if possible, from a specialist in elder law. Figure out the health care necessities for your loved one in the short, middle, and long-term, and any matters regarding their money and properties. There are healthcare options such as Medicare, Medicaid, and special programs for veterans.

Inform your family that you're consulting a lawyer, and offer them the chance to attend the meeting if they want to. This is already a delicate situation, and seeing a lawyer behind your family's back could generate unnecessary conflict. Even if they can't be there, offer the lawyer a list of names, addresses, emails, and telephone numbers of all family members who wish to be involved.

Make sure that you bring all the documents to your appointment with the lawyer. You will need copies of recent income taxes returns, of real estate deeds, and of estate planning documents, such as trusts and wills. Bring also copies of health, life, and long-term care insurance policies, including their cash values. A list of assets is also helpful, including bank accounts, vehicles, and real estate, with details about their current value and the names of the owners, account holders, and beneficiaries.

Be thorough when preparing these documents. It can be a stressful process, but it's better to bring more than you need than too little. Otherwise, you could create an uncertainty between your family members later on, leaving space for them to question who actually has a voice in decision-making regarding the dementia patient.

Your lawyer will prepare a document called power of attorney, which legally establishes who will be in charge of taking care of the dementia patient when they can no longer make their own decisions, including financial decisions. That person is usually a spouse or a child, and they become the primary caregiver. In case they are not able to fulfill that role, the lawyer should name a successor agent.

A power of attorney becomes valid at the stage of dementia in which the person cannot be trusted to make their own decisions. A doctor should evaluate when they have reached that state, by which point the designated agent takes charge of their finances and other business. The agent is expected to make all decisions in the best interest of the dementia patient.

The power of attorney agent is also expected to take care of matters regarding the healthcare of the dementia patient. They may or may not be the same person who takes care of the finances and are designated by a document known as advance directive. It's their responsibility to choose the methods of treatment and care settings and to choose the doctors that fit their loved one's necessity. They are also responsible for end-of-life decisions, which allows the dementia patient to die with dignity and to take care of funeral arrangements.

The lawyer will also assist the dementia patient in creating a will. This is a document that becomes valid after the person's death and appoints a person to manage the estate and the people who will receive the assets in that estate—the executor and the beneficiaries, respectively. The authority of these people only becomes valid once the person dies.

Without a power of attorney, you might have to establish a guardianship or conservatorship when the dementia patient has progressed to a stage where they lack legal capacity. This involves a court proceeding where a judge appoints a guardian or conservator to make decisions on behalf of the person with dementia. The process of becoming a guardian can be long, as there are different laws in that regard from state to state. The guardian's job is to make decisions regarding the health and financial situation of the person with dementia and also assist them with their activities of daily living.

A living trust is a legal document that establishes a grantor who will distribute a person's assets after their demise. The grantor will designate a trustee, which can be an individual or an entity, to control that distribution. This document helps to avoid fights and legal processes between the family members, which can go on for a long time and generate conflict.

One of the most important documents that a dementia patient can use to have their desires respected is a living will. With this document, the patients specify what treatments they allow to be used to keep them alive and which ones are not acceptable. They also state their wishes regarding organ donation and pain management. Through a living will, the patient can say yes or no to dialysis, mechanical ventilation, or tube feeding.

People with severe illnesses can also use a document called portable medical order (POLST) to inform what kind of medical assistance they want to receive later on. Again, each state has its own laws regarding this document, and you need to ask for a form from your healthcare provider. Once the form is filled out, it will be included in the person's medical records, so all doctors who take care of them in the future will know it.

PLANNING FOR MONEY

Dementia is an expensive condition, and you need to plan how you are going to handle the costs in the future. The disease comes without warning, but there are things you can do in advance that will make all the difference. As we've seen, dementia isn't a normal part of growing old, but you can assume that your aging relatives are subject to having it, and it wouldn't hurt you to take some precautions.

As you help your loved one plan for their retirement, it's wise to include the possibility of needing care for dementia. Talk to a financial adviser, and figure out how much your loved one would need to live with dignity during the several stages of the disease. Their retirement income may not be enough, in which case you might have to talk to other relatives to establish a fund for that purpose. If dementia strikes, you'll be covered. If it doesn't, all the better!

Maybe you don't have time for that anymore. Your loved one has already shown signs of dementia, and you didn't establish the fund to take care of them. An important step is to designate someone to take care of the money and assets that your loved one has in their savings account or in a bank. Consider drawing up a consent agreement or adding yourself to your loved one's banking account to help them manage money once they can't.

Please don't add multiple people because money can vanish, and no one will admit to anything.

Getting long-term care insurance services will also make a difference in the treatment. This kind of insurance offers several services that are not included in traditional health insurance, including care that can be offered at the patient's home, a nursing home, an assisted living facility, or an adult day care center.

CHAPTER 2 PRACTICAL EXERCISE

Here's a checklist of legal matters regarding dementia. Mark the ones you've already accomplished.

- Initiating a conversation while the dementia person is still capable of expressing their desires and understands the consequences of their decisions.
- Finding a licensed attorney to take care of legal matters.
- Locate and secure all legal documents (wills, trusts, contacts, etc.) your loved one has entered into no less than five years prior to their diagnosis.
- The patient should prepare a living will and outline their wishes regarding medical treatments they want to receive or not receive if they are unable to communicate or make decisions.
- They should also write a will with their wishes regarding the management and disposal of a person's estate during their life and after death.
- Get a power of attorney, a legal document appointing someone else to make decisions on the dementia patient's behalf.
- Keep the family informed of all these negotiations.

One person caring for another represents life's greatest value.

— JIM COHN

Family conflicts and suspicions will increase your self-doubt if you let them. Believe in your capacity and that you're the right person to guide the person you love through this journey. It's all about the rights and needs of your loved one. Other people will have their opinion, but they don't know what it's like to be in your shoes.

Estranged families often come together with the common mission of taking care of a loved one with dementia. Everyone can put their differences aside, abandon long-time grudges, and give their best together. In other cases, the differences might be too large to forget, whether the issue is with the caregiver, or the person being taken care of. While dementia erases memories and personality traits from those who are suffering from it, their faults may continue to be alive in the hearts of those around them.

As a caregiver, your job is to put all of that aside and do the best job you can with the tools and help you have. You'll find that time is precious and that you can't spend your energy trying to convince others to help. While all this happens, it helps to move into chapter three to understand what you can expect after your loved one's diagnosis.

3

WHAT YOU CAN EXPECT AFTER
THE DIAGNOSIS

You and your family may have been trying to prepare yourselves for the diagnosis for a few months, going back and forth with doctors and watching your loved one decline. There are many exams needed, and you hope it's just an age thing, something that happens to every elderly person. You have been doing some research of your own, looking on the internet and reading books such as this one. Then, the doctor calls you into their office and gives the final diagnosis. Your loved one has dementia.

Take this opportunity to ask the doctor every question you might have about how dementia works. Ask them for his card and the cards of every professional that can be helpful in this situation. That includes clinics and therapists that can attend to your loved one, but also people who can help you with your mental health as this situation progresses. You are an important part of that process and can't afford to have a breakdown.

33

Each part of the brain handles a distinct part of a person's body functions, habits, and memories. When these cells die, the signs of dementia appear. You will notice that the person is saying and doing unusual things and not acting like themselves. The kind of dementia depends on what part of the brain is losing neurons (brain cells). As the signs and symptoms of dementia progress, you might feel lost without understanding what's happening to your loved one. There is a medical reason behind the emotional state and change of behavior of a dementia patient, and it's important to know how that works.

A dementia patient may have difficulty following conversations, responding to their environment, and remembering people around them, which causes anger and frustration. Stimuli such as noises and lights that feel natural to people around them can be overbearing to the dementia patient.

Pain caused by infections and other medical issues can cause a change in behavior, especially if they can't express it. Beware that, even in a person who has been diagnosed with dementia, the dementia itself may not be the cause for changing behavior. This could be a way for your loved one to pass you a message. They might not transmit their fear, confusion, or other over-whelming sensations in any other way and resort to being angry and irritated. If the behavior continues, take them to a GP to have them examined.

Some people make the mistake of dismissing this behavior, thinking it's a mere whim of an old person wanting attention. However, this behavior can become risky and hazardous if the person walks out of their house on their own. While you can deal with annoying and frustrating behavior with soft manners, risky and hazardous behavior requires a stronger response, such as installing alarms at the door.

We are now going to explore the different parts of the brain.

Frontal Lobe

The frontal lobe is located directly behind your forehead. This part of the brain handles behavior and personality, emotions, self-control, judgment, thinking, muscle control, muscle movements, and memory storage. It also provides the ability to multi-task and maintain short-term memory. Since the frontal lobe handles higher executive functions, people with frontotemporal dementia first show changes in their personalities.

People with damaged frontal lobes have a short attention span and find it difficult to concentrate. It's hard for them to find a narrative, find motivation, and complete tasks they were used to doing by themselves. The passiveness and lack of interaction in the first stages of frontal lobe damage are replaced by impulsiveness and disinhibition as the neurons continue to die, which could lead the person to improper public behavior.

Parietal Lobe

The parietal lobe is at the top rear of your head, under the crown of the skull. It's responsible for sensory perception and integration, managing touch, temperature, pressure, pain, and your five senses—vision, hearing, touch, smell, and taste. The parietal lobe is also responsible for two-point discrimination, the ability to discern two different objects touching our skin as more than one.

People with damage to their parietal lobe find it hard to express themselves through words. You will notice that they avoid social interactions and conversations because of their frustration with not finding words. This leads to irritation and confusion with the environment, making them agitated and prone to wandering.

Temporal Lobe

The two temporal lobes are behind the ears in each brain hemisphere and are separated from the frontal lobe by a lateral fissure. Their job is to process sensory information, allowing you to interact with the world around you, recognize language, process emotions, and form and access memories.

Frontotemporal dementia is rare and often happens to people between 45 to 64 years old (*What Are Frontotemporal Disorders? Causes, Symptoms, and Treatment*, n.d.-b), and it attacks the frontal global as well as the temporal lobes. Symptoms include emotional problems, unusual behavior, and difficulty walking, working, and communicating.

Occipital Lobe

At the back of the head, the occipital lobe is responsible for visuospatial processing and memory formation. It has the primary visual cortex, which processes the information sent by the eyes, generating distance and depth perception, color determination, object and face recognition.

Occipital lobe dementia makes it difficult for the person to see what's in front of them, causing issues with coordination, memory loss, confusion, blurred and double vision, and difficulty recognizing objects or faces.

THE EMOTIONAL IMPACT OF DEMENTIA

Being diagnosed with dementia can generate a rollercoaster of emotions, especially if you don't have enough information about the disease. Some people get despaired, angry, shocked, and scared, while others surprise those around them—and themselves—by being cool and rational about it. After months or even years of not knowing what's wrong with you, it's rewarding to know that your condition has a name and treatment.

That's not most cases, though, and hearing the d-word from a doctor often throws people into depression and anxiety. People around them should be there to help them cope with those emotions and deal with their own thoughts and feelings about the struggle that lies ahead.

A dementia patient can be emotionally unpredictable, having peaks of emotion and changes in mood, being irritable and grumpy at one moment and warm and joyful at the next. You will notice they get lost in conversations and are often uninterested in things that once fascinated them.

Dealing with these peaks isn't easy, but remember they are caused by the progressive death of neurons in your loved one's brain. Also, don't think that they will not notice these changes— they can be as frustrating and annoying to you as they are to them, even if they don't recognize it rationally.

Instead of getting angry and talking back to your loved one, try to understand what's behind their behavior. You'll often find that they are asking for help in the only way they know how. If, for example, they get agitated and nervous when you're taking them to the toilet, that could be their way of telling you they have a urinary infection and are experiencing pain.

A dementia patient is losing contact with the world around them. They see their senses, thoughts, memories, and words escaping their mind. That leads to insecurity and loss of self-confidence. Even in cases in which the family decides not to tell them about their condition, they can tell there's something different in the way people treat them, which affects their mood and behavior.

You might try your best to take care of your loved one and feel that they are not responding in the way you expected. The most basic thing you can do is not to lose your temper. Praise minor achievements, such as finishing a meal by themselves, and avoid being overly critical of their mistakes. Even the smallest enjoyment will make a difference in their mind. Take them outside to enjoy the sun and fresh air, offer them company when they watch TV, and laugh with them. You'll see that your own mind will benefit from it.

Poor mental health can exaggerate dementia symptoms. A dementia patient should be kept away from stressful situations, such as excessive noise, and avoid information that could harm their serenity. It's difficult to diagnose depression in a dementia patient since their symptoms are intertwined. Poor sleep, lack of energy and interest, confusion, loss of appetite, emotional turmoil, and feelings of worthlessness and sadness are all symptoms related to both conditions.

The same doctor who diagnosed dementia in your loved one can prescribe antidepressant medication to improve their mood, appetite, sleep, and willingness to take part in activities. The doctor will also explain the side effects of those antidepressants before starting the treatment. A medicine that does wonders for the brain but causes side effects such as headaches, nausea, and shaking should be discontinued.

Knowing each treatment has its limitations will save you from frustration. You should also know your own limitations and not push yourself to your own breakdown. Don't put all of your hopes into a miraculous medicine that promises to restore the mental health of your loved one, and don't treat them as if it's their fault for being like that—as if they are not trying hard enough to get better.

CHANGES TO COME

You will be a better caregiver if you know what lies ahead. It's important to keep in mind that memory loss caused by dementia isn't the same as the one caused by healthy aging. While an aging person may forget their keys or someone's name, the dementia patient suffers constant memory loss, to the point they can't live normally anymore. This memory loss is progressive, meaning it only gets worse with time and develops into the most basic actions, such as washing or dressing.

The information that a dementia patient stores over their lives, whether historical, cultural, or political, will fade away. It's also common to mix dates and facts, for example, placing themselves into a historical event in which they were not present. Following the story of a movie or TV show also becomes difficult, and they will pay more attention to the immediate aspects of the image and sound rather than following the plot and characters. Another aspect in which they suffer is following verbal directions to arrive at a place, even if that place is inside their own house.

Some cases of dementia come with hallucinations and delusions, which feel very real to the person who's suffering from them. This can have a devastating influence on their condition. They may see monsters and boogeymen from their childhood, sense a disaster, or panic when they don't recognize their face in a mirror.

Telling your loved one that what they're seeing isn't real may not be enough. You might have to take them to a doctor and get them treated with antipsychotic medication. This kind of medicine comes with side effects, which are milder in the more modern ones.

You should not confirm the hallucinations your loved one is sensing, but you can acknowledge they are confused and that you are going to find a solution to that problem together. Ask them simple questions, even if you already know the answers, and that will help you guide them through this situation. If, for example, they insist they are in the wrong house and that they want to go home, you can go along with it and say that you are taking a vacation together at that place.

Like other behaviors, hallucinations are often signs that your loved one is trying to say something. In some cases, you will have to investigate their origin and find out if there's something real about them. When they scream about an evil entity hurting them, they might talk about someone who had physically abused them when you were not watching.

Memory loss in the later stages of dementia has an extreme effect on recent memories. By then, the dementia patient won't remember events of the same day, such as what they had for lunch. Older memories will also be affected, and the dementia patient may believe they're living in another moment of their lives. They may believe they're paying a visit to someone else's house when in fact, they are in their own house where they've lived for years.

It's common for people at that stage to confuse their loved ones with someone else. For example, they may think that the daughter who's caring for them is their mother or that their spouse is a stranger in their house. Trying to make them remember people's identity isn't easy. Many times, even if they don't know who someone is, their feelings for that person can remain, and sometimes that's what matters. You can experiment with introducing yourself again each time you see them, but be prepared to be forgotten right after.

Even as their mind fades away, people with dementia can find interest in fun and enjoyable activities as long as they are adapted to their mental conditions. Someone who enjoyed playing chess before dementia may not engage in that game anymore, but you can find simpler and more colorful board games that will capture their attention. You can also stimulate them through their senses with the touch of a soft blanket, the feel of a hand lotion, or the satisfying motions of a sensory toddler game.

Aphasia

Aphasia is a communication disorder that makes people use the wrong words during a conversation. If your loved one is having trouble recalling common words, such as objects in front of them, and calling them by a different name, it can be because of their dementia. Aphasia also causes people to mistake the name of people close to them.

Problems With Movement

People with dementia may fall, trip, and slip often. This kind of movement issue is caused by a difficulty of interacting with their surroundings and poses a danger to their safety. It helps if they shuffle their legs while walking instead of lifting them from the ground.

Problems With Sight

In some rare cases, dementia can affect sight, even in people with healthy eyes. People with dementia can also lose the ability to read the hours in an analog clock. That could also be because of a difficulty with dealing with numbers, which is a problem that also hinders them from following instructions and keeping control of their money.

Problems With Sleep

Older people have a tendency to lose sleep quality, but it's worse for people with dementia. Falling and staying asleep can be an issue, as they get agitated at bedtime. They may also wake up in the middle of the night and want to start their day while it's still dark. That insomnia is related to dementia risk factors, but also to behavioral issues and can be caused by the death of their neurons, excessive medication, a diet with lots of sugar and caffeine, or the use of electronic screens before going to bed.

Hoarding

Dementia can lead to hoarding as a response to isolation and the feeling of losing things. Old things may bring them back to a moment in the past and they may also declare precious things are missing. Help them to be more organized and take the time to assist them in finding each object that they declare missing.

Delirium

A sudden change of behavior or fast decrease of mental abilities could be caused by delirium. You will notice that the person is muttering gibberish or expressing strange ideas, being unable to concentrate, having hallucinations and delusions, and not following their regular sleeping cycle. This situation requires medical help.

Repetitions

Verbal repetitions are common in people with dementia. They repeat statements and questions to the point that it becomes annoying for the caregiver and other people around them. When the same answer doesn't satisfy them, you can offer a distraction, such as going for a walk or offering food they like. Issues with motor behaviors are also common, which can be caused by their difficulties in expressing their needs and emotions.

Wandering

Leaving dementia patients by themselves, even for a short amount of time, can cause them to wander. Sixty percent of patients wander (Hobson, 2023b), which can pose a threat to their safety. They may wander because of too much energy, boredom, discomfort, or pain. They might also relive the past, walking along a route they used to take, or going to visit someone that may not be there anymore. In some cases, they acquire aberrant motor behavior, fidgeting and wringing their hands and clothes.

Sundowning

Late afternoon and early evening can be a hard time for people with dementia, who show signs of anxiety, insecurity, or confusion as it begins to darken—a disorder known as sundowning. As their disoriented behavior becomes difficult, they might suffer hallucinations. You'll notice that they feel restless and upset, affecting their concentration and attention span. This can be treated with medication, and it helps if you offer them some kind of distraction during that period of the day.

Aggression

Cases of physical and aggressive behavior from the dementia patient have to be dealt with using extreme care. If they escalate, they can be a serious threat to the caregiver and other loved ones. Insults and threats may not sound as harmful as physical assault, but they are all forms of violence. This kind of behavior may come out of nowhere, even from peaceful patients. It can be a way for them to manifest their fear or frustration, as it's often caused by loud noises and physical clutter.

It's imperative that you keep calm during aggressions, try to find the origin of their anxiety, and remove it when possible. Sometimes the cause of the aggression is clear and palpable, such as loud music or strong light. In other cases, it's caused by a physical discomfort that only a doctor can find and treat.

Anxiety

Anxiety is one of the most common symptoms of dementia, affecting 71% of the patients (Tee-Melegrito, 2022). Unable to process and adapt to new stimuli and information, the dementia patient has a constant feeling of inadequacy, leading them to feel anxious. They may also lose interest in their daily activities, making them apathetic and depressed.

Loss of Filters

As they lose contact with social norms, your loved ones may show inappropriate behavior, such as making sexual comments, removing their clothes in public, or going to the bathroom in public. This can also manifest itself in less extreme ways, such as losing table manners and disrespecting others. Talk to your family and friends about this behavior, so they can be prepared for it, and keep your loved one away from places that can trigger that kind of behavior.

Psychosis

Some dementia patients develop psychosis, in which the person becomes involuntarily agitated and incoherent, though experts still don't understand why. Psychosis affects memory and the ability to recognize and process new information, especially visual information. It also causes hallucinations and illusions, making the person doubt their beliefs and sense things that don't exist.

METHODS TO HANDLE BEHAVIOR CHANGES

One of the most challenging aspects of being a caregiver comes when your loved one doesn't seem to act like themselves anymore. As brain cells die, you may feel like it's a different person in their body. As we've seen, the death of neurons in different parts of the brain causes distinct changes in behaviors since each lobe handles different aspects of brain function.

The impact of dementia extends to environmental perception and to the interactions between the person who's affected and those who try to understand what's going on inside their minds. Also, don't underestimate the role that pain and discomfort play in this change of behavior. Just as a baby screams and cries when they're hungry, or their diapers are dirty, the dementia patient will ask for help using the tools they still have.

Look for what's triggering the change of behavior, which can be related to something from the person's past. People with dementia are sensitive to abrupt changes in their normal routine, such as an unwanted visit. Pay attention to how they act when they are around certain people. If they get agitated and nervous when someone is around, there might be a reason for that.

A change of behavior poses a hazard to the patient's security if, for example, they hurt themselves with metal forks and knives. Replacing them with plastic ones won't solve the entire problem, but it is a safer alternative. In other cases, the behavior is just frustrating and annoying, such as throwing their food on the ground which requires patience and care, even when the person keeps repeating it.

You need to earn the confidence of the dementia patient. This isn't easy, and every caregiver goes through that awful moment when they just want to scream at their loved one's faces. This could have disastrous consequences. Instead, train yourself to accept what they are going through rather than what they are. If you can, do a little breathing exercise, drink a glass of water, count to ten, then go back to work.

A structured and predictable routine will benefit not only the dementia patient but also you, the caregiver. Dementia is an unpredictable condition, and you won't always be able to follow the plan. But having a plan will help you navigate through each part of the day, from the moment you wake up the dementia patient through their meals, baths, and walks, ending when you put them into bed.

Remember that you are not alone, and there are many other caregivers going through the same difficulties as you. They may live in your neighborhood, your street, or even in your building, and getting in contact with them will help you carry your burden and learn more about what you're doing.

The DICE system is great for navigating through the harshest stages of dementia. It stands for Describe, Investigate, Create, and Evaluate, and it helps you and your loved one to manage your behavior skills. Here's how it goes:

D: Describe What Happens

Patient

- What is the patient doing?
- How is the patient reacting?
- Is the patient a threat to their own security?

Caregiver

- How is the patient's behavior affecting your mind?
- How is the patient's behavior affecting your safety?
- Are you being affected mentally or physically by their behavior?
- What's your response?

Environment

- What were the environmental conditions before the behavior occurred?
- At what time did the behavior occur, and was it related to a specific activity?
- Where did the behavior take place?
- What events preceded the behavior? What happened after it?

I: Investigate Possible Causes

Patient

- Has the patient's medication been changed recently?
- Is the patient incapable of doing things?
- Is there any previous medical condition that may be affecting the patient?

- What are the patient's unmet needs? Are they hungry, thirsty, bored, constipated, overwhelmed, etc.?
- What mental health issues are affecting the patient?
- Is the patient hearing or sight impaired?
- Does the patient have memory problems or cognitive impairment?
- Is the patient afraid or embarrassed?

Caregiver

- What aspects of the situation aren't you considering?
- Can the patient be suffering for something you've ignored?
- Could you use a different approach in this situation?
- Do you have realistic expectations regarding what the patient can do?
- Can you identify other stressors or mood issues in this situation?
- Can family or cultural issues be affecting your client?

Environment

- Is the environment overstimulating the patient?
- Is the environment under stimulating the patient?
- Is the environment around the patient disorienting or lacking visual clues?
- How stiff is the routine, and could it benefit from small changes?
- Is the patient being offered activities and tasks that use their abilities and garner their interest?

C: Create a Plan

Patient

- Develop a response to the patient's unfulfilled needs.
- Suspend high-risk medications.
- Take them to their primary care provider to discuss potential medical causes.
- Improve mental health treatment.
- Get them used to activity during the day and rest at night.

Caregiver

- Look for support and information.
- Be more communicative.
- Offer activities that improve quality of life.
- Keep your tasks simple.
- Take care of yourself.
- Look for help, whether from professionals or from family and friends.
- Assess potential safety risks and take practical steps to prevent them.

Environment

- Make sure the environment is safe and simple by removing clutter.
- Choose the best environment for each activity.
- Create an environment that's visually interesting, with pictures, labels, and color contrast.
- Select a place to keep your important things, such as keys, phones, wallets, and important documents.
- Make the environment accessible.

E: Evaluate the Plan

Patient

- What were the changes in treatments and strategies?
- Which changes worked, and which didn't.
- Has the patient experienced side effects?

Caregiver

- What did you try? How helpful was each action?
- Do you feel there's room to try new things?

Environment

- What did you try? How helpful was each action?
- Do you feel there's room to try new things?

THE 6 R'S OF BEHAVIORAL MANAGEMENT

The Johns Hopkins Health Alert offers *The 6 R's of Managing Difficult Behavior From the 36-Hour Day* (2010), based on the research of Peter Rabins, M.D. and Nancy Mace, which help to deal with difficulties regarding people with dementia. It's divided into six main steps:

1. restriction
2. reassess
3. reconsider
4. rechannel
5. reassure
6. review

These take into consideration the many frustrations, embarrassments, and dangers that caregivers have to go through. That includes hazardous and non-hazardous behavior, both of which can damage the quality of life of everyone involved. The challenge here is to deal with these issues while still doing a good job at taking care of the dementia patient.

Restriction is the most basic dementia strategy, and it involves stopping the dementia patient from conducting that behavior. That may involve force, which isn't ideal, but it might be necessary to stop them from hurting someone or themselves.

Reassess is dementia strategy #2. It involves identifying if a physical problem, such as pain, an infection, an itch, or anything of the sort that might be behind a change of behavior. A triggering noise, fatigue, insomnia, and sundowning are other causes of agitation.

Reconsider is dementia strategy #3, and it's about putting yourself in the shoes of the dementia patient. By trying to think like them, you can figure out what's happening, how frustrating their situation is, and what part the environment plays in that agitation.

Rechannel is dementia strategy #4, in which you acknowledge the agitation and try to make it less disruptive to the dementia patient. You can replace breakable objects with rubber toys that they can throw around without making a mess and also involves hiding important objects in safe places so they can't hide or destroy them.

Reassure is dementia strategy #5, and it's simply a matter of comforting the dementia patient when their frustration results in fear, anger, or anxiety. Let them know you are there for them and that the environment is safe.

Review is dementia strategy #6, and it's more directed to the caregiver than the patient. After an episode in which you needed to employ some or all of the strategies above, you should review your performance and figure out what you could have done better the next time.

THE WANT MODEL

The WANT model, presented by Wang (2022), defends that people with dementia always assume behavioral and psychological symptoms of dementia (BPSD) because they can't meet physiological, mental, emotional, and social needs. There's an unbalance between personal traits and environment, which is aggravated by dementia.

Neurological and cognitive aspects also play a role in these behaviors, as well as their overall health, disabilities, and emotional status. Psychosocial factors can't be dismissed since they will play a role in the treatment that the patient gets. Surely a wealthy person will have access to better treatment and medical care than someone living on welfare.

The unmet needs that cause BPSD have a lot to do with the surroundings where the person is living, in turn, bringing up old personality traits and habits. The many issues caused by dementia can take the patient's mind back to when they were out of control in their life, had problems with health, or lost loved ones. They try to connect with the outside world, which results in BPSDs as a way of asking the caregiver to give them some safety and structure.

CHAPTER 3 PRACTICAL EXERCISE

You are now going to use the DICE method and apply it to the loved one you're taking care of. Start small by identifying one of their disruptive behaviors—the one that bothers you the most—and analyze it through the points that we mentioned earlier in this chapter.

For example, if your loved one has memory problems that cause them to misplace items, you can write what objects have been missing, where they were found, and which ones disappeared for good. Knowing the objects, how they went missing, and where they were placed will help you understand how that behavior works.

It's embarrassing when your loved one takes their clothes off in public, but the solution isn't to seclude them inside the house. To find the proper solution, you need to investigate why and when they take their clothes off and what kind of need they are trying to meet. This is crucial for you to create and apply a plan that will help that kind of behavior go away.

Once you identify one of these behaviors and pass them through the four stages of the DICE System, you'll see that the solution may be simpler than you imagined. You don't have to answer all the bullet points on that list every time you do this exercise, but it helps to take all of them into consideration. You may find out things that you'd never imagine otherwise.

 Some days, there won't be a song in your heart. Sing anyway.

— EMORY AUSTIN

Embracing your loved one or patient's behavioral or personality changes will temporarily remove your heart's song, but don't stop singing. You understand much more than you did an hour ago. By now, you know that the dementia patient assumes certain behaviors when they feel there's something wrong within them or when they feel out of place or threatened by their environment. Rather than repressing them, you need to understand what's wrong and do your best to fix it.

In these first three chapters, we've seen plenty of theory, which is necessary to form a base of knowledge. Now, it's time to do what you must to support your loved one. In the next chapters, you'll learn the practical side of being a caregiver and how to apply the concepts we've seen so far into action.

4

CHOOSING A SUPPORT NETWORK FOR YOUR LOVED ONE

*Y*ou are not supposed to fight this fight alone. There's no shame in looking for help, inside and outside the family, and dividing your responsibility with others. It's time to build the tribe of professionals, friends, and supporters you both need on this journey.

Social interactions are essential for people with dementia. People, friends, and family can shy away because of dementia's challenging behaviors and symptoms. However, social interactions are a must, and you'll get them through friendly and caregiving support.

CHOOSING THE RIGHT DOCTOR

It's never easy for an older person to switch doctors. That might be necessary, though, if the doctor they're used to can't assist with their care any longer or if they are not qualified to deal with dementia. They may offer some resistance to going to a new doctor, but if that's necessary, there are a few ways of making that easier.

The first aspect to consider while choosing a doctor to take care of your loved one is their accessibility. You may find a great doctor who you get along with but whose office is in another town. That won't do. You also need to check their working hours and how easily you can get an appointment. Give preference to those who are available during evenings, weekends, and holidays.

The first appointment is crucial, and you should make it before your loved one begins to deteriorate. The goal here is to introduce yourself and your loved one to the new physician and see if the three of you get along and can trust each other. Some practices offer this first consultation for free. The doctor will ask you about the medications your loved one is on, and it helps to write the list down or to bring the medicines with you.

Consider also how well-equipped the doctor's lab is and whether they can conduct important exams by themselves instead of sending you to a lab. You will find practices that offer more than one medical service, and it's great to have all you need at the same address. Their staff should be well trained and qualified to deal with dementia patients without losing their composure. Finding a practice that has these features and also accepts your insurance isn't easy, but it's possible.

Doctors are there to provide you with a service, and you can and should ask them questions. Pay attention to the answers, and you'll notice if they like to talk about themselves. For example, if you ask them what their greatest strengths are, they might talk about their discipline, motivation, and ability to take action. Ask them how much time they like to spend with each patient, and follow up with what they want for you. Another tricky question you can ask is how they would act if you brought a diagnosis you found on the internet to debunk their opinion. Doctors hate it when you do that, and this is a good way of checking their patience. Finish your questioning by asking them if they have anything to ask you.

Whenever you see a change of behavior in your loved one, take them to their primary care doctor. They will examine them to determine if the change is caused by a physical or mental issue, and conduct brief memory-screening tests to evaluate their mental state. They will decide if the patient needs the help of a specialist, and will work together with them to help with the diagnosis.

Primary care doctors often have experience with older people, but you need one who also has experience with different forms of dementia. Neurologists are trained to take care of dementia cases but there are also specialists, such as geriatricians, geriatric nurse practitioners, and geriatric psychiatrists, who have special skills while dealing with older people.

Seeking recommendations from other caregivers will save you time and legwork. You can also seek help in local hospitals and senior centers, as well as organizations such as the National Association of Area Agencies on Aging and the Alzheimer's Association, which offers a Community Resource Finder page. A doctor who works great for your neighbor with Alzheimer's may not serve the needs of your loved one with vascular dementia, but it's a start.

As much as you try to be with your loved one at every appointment, that's not always possible. You need to find out how everything went from the person who went in your place. Instruct them to take notes at the appointment, and even write a report detailing each step. If that's not enough, call the doctor's office and ask all the questions you need.

To talk to your doctor about your loved one's condition, you may need a HIPAA authorization, a document that expresses the dementia patient's consent to use or disclose their protected health information. You may also need a power of attorney document signed by a lawyer. These documents are not always necessary, but it's better to have them on hand to avoid issues.

Be honest to your loved one about where you're taking them and what they can expect during their appointment. Let them know that you'll be by their side to advocate for their health, and that they should trust you during this process.

Arriving at the office, have a private word with the doctor about the behavior of your loved one, and the tricks they might try during the appointment. Another way of doing that is to call beforehand, or send the doctor an email about the kind of behavior, so they can be prepared. It would be useful to you if you could—and you should—write in a diary about the dementia patient's behavior, attach that to the email, and that information will be valuable to the doctor.

A dementia patient requires a doctor who's warm and interested. If your doctor just stares at the screen of their computer and offers you prescriptions, it might be a good idea to look for someone else. You are trying to build a relationship between you, your loved one, and the person who's supposed to take care of their health. When that doesn't work, the whole treatment plan is jeopardized.

Older people sometimes lie to the doctors in fear of facing their situation. They know there's something wrong with them, and don't want to have that fear materialized in a diagnosis. Knowing they have a disease means losing control over themselves, which could lead them to underplay their symptoms, or pretend they're okay. This isn't always conscious, and could come from a sense of denial regarding their own health. Deep down they feel that if they don't talk about what's wrong, it will make it disappear.

Pretending that they're okay can be exhausting to aging patients, but some of them try to put on a show to pretend that they are 100% okay, a phenomenon known as show-timing. At home they may have trouble remembering what they ate for lunch, only to arrive at the doctor's office and improvise a menu on top of their head. That serves for physical issues as well. A patient who has trouble standing up because of bad knees can hide their pain during the appointment to pretend everything is alright.

Having a doctor who's involved at each step of the treatment will make a difference. They not only need to inform you of what kind of dementia your loved one has and how far they are in the treatment, but also guide you during the next steps. They need to be honest to you, without pretending this is going to be easy, while also being reassuring and present but also advising you about what is coming.

GETTING A NURSE

Family members are the most common caregivers for people with dementia, but their lack of experience can be a problem. Hiring a professional nurse can be expensive, but it will provide your loved one with the specialized care they need during the different stages of dementia. Mild and moderate cases of dementia may not require a professional nurse, but hiring one early on will help to create a relationship between you, the nurse, and the patient, which will be helpful later on.

More extensive nursing care is advisable during moderate and advanced stages of dementia, when patients have the risk of falling, have trouble speaking, and need help with hygiene. A nurse is also trained to be patient and offer compassion and care in a way that untrained people aren't. Even a loving son or daughter may get impatient by repetitive behavior from the dementia patient, while the nurse is trained to deal with that.

Make sure your nurse follows proper nursing procedures, paying attention to what you hear and see throughout the visit and taking notes about it. That won't turn you into a professional, but it can be helpful when they're not around. Certain tasks, such as tube feeding the patient when they cannot do it, require formal training.

The risk of choking happens not only when the patient is eating but also when they take their medicines. The nurse should administer the medicine in those situations, and also when the patient requires an IV injection. Your loved one might require different medications during different times of the day, so if possible, arrange for the nurse to be there at those times—the ideal is to have different nurses attending 24 hours a day in shifts.

An ideal nurse should be patient, compassionate, and caring. Having excellent communication skills with people suffering from dementia makes a difference. The dementia patient often isn't fond of the nurse and gets agitated at their presence. It's common for patients to claim that the nurse is trying to harm them and not want to take the medicine. Some will go to the extreme by hiding a pill under their tongue and spit it when the nurse isn't around. It's the nurse's job to observe such situations and deal with them appropriately.

People with dementia don't act that way just because they're petty. Their cognitive functions are impaired by the damage to their brain, which affects their decision making and personality. Seeing a stranger enter their lives, in such a close relationship is scary since they can't express their feelings effectively. They feel annoyed, misunderstood, and even threatened, and become physically aggressive by punching, kicking, and biting. A professional nurse can understand all of that and handle the aggression, while doing what needs to be done. If a pill must be administered to that patient, the nurse will achieve that without violence and without getting their feelings hurt.

A good way of looking for a nurse is by contacting your local Alzheimer's Association chapter and asking for referrals. You can also contact services such as an eldercare locator, which can provide you with a nurse at any time of the day. Your personal doctor should also be able to recommend competent nurses.

Interviewing a nurse is a serious business. You need to ask them about their experience with dementia patients, and verify if they have dealt with all the different stages of the disease. That experience should have shown them what kind of dementia patients they're most suited for. Ask about their communication skills with people suffering from dementia, and how they feel about the environment where they're going to work. By the end of the interview, you should understand their professional philosophy and their idea of what it takes to be a good nurse.

GERIATRIC CARE MANAGER

If you're having trouble meeting all the needs of your loved one suffering from dementia, consider hiring the services of a geriatric care manager. This is a resourceful professional who will help you develop a strategy so you can hire the best professionals and make the right decisions.

A geriatric care manager will help you figure out a long-term care plan, talking you through the most complex topics, managing medical services, and evaluating the needs of your home environment. This isn't a cheap service and isn't covered by insurance. However, it can be crucial for families who live far apart and can't all be there at the same time for the dementia patient.

A licensed geriatric manager should have a nursing or social assistant background. Make sure they have education and experience before hiring them, and don't be afraid to ask for their references. They should be able to provide home care services, communicate all information with you, and be around whenever you need them.

THE SOCIAL LIFE OF A DEMENTIA PATIENT

Having dementia doesn't mean forsaking one's social life. As the disease progresses, it's important for your loved one to be near people and engage in activities they enjoy. Staying close to family and friends brings many benefits, and it can make a big difference during the late stages of the disease. Their personality will have changed by then, and they may not remember the names of people around them.

A social structure will help them avoid feeling alone and lost, daydreaming inside their head. As they socialize, the dementia patient is reminded of the names of people, places, and things, which increases their awareness capabilities. It also keeps their mind in the present, rather than going back and forth in their memories and getting lost in wandering thoughts.

Different people experience their own kind of loneliness. It's possible to be lonely while surrounded by people, and be comfortable when away from everyone. Before introducing your loved one to new people see how they interact with those who they already know. Are they able to focus on the present during a conversation, or is their mind wandering even when you're talking about a subject that interests them?

It's possible to exercise the brain through socialization. A strong brain is more resistant to the effects of dementia. But, just as you can't ask a person to lift a 40 lb. weight on the first day at the gym, you shouldn't overstimulate the brain. Be careful not to overwhelm the dementia patient with too much social interaction. Crowding their personal space with too many people can overstimulate their senses, which leads to stress and anxiety. The effect is the opposite of the desirable and may lead them to social phobia.

A dementia patient can feel they're losing control of their mind, even if they don't know or can't remember their diagnosis. That leads to anger and frustration, not at a specific person, but at the effects that dementia has on their minds. Socializing will keep their mind distracted from their condition and in their interaction with people they enjoy. This leads to a feeling of self-worth, which keeps them happier.

A dementia patient needs to be in a friendly environment. That means more than having a fall-proof house—you also need to keep them away from their emotional triggers. Sometimes you can only learn what those are when they affect your loved one, and even in that situation, they may be hard to understand. You may have had a neighbor for years, but out of nowhere, their current presence caused panic attacks for your loved one. Have a friendly conversation and try to find out about what triggered them. They may mix different stories in their head, but your job here isn't to correct them, but to be patient and to know what to do.

During the COVID-19 pandemic, socializing became even harder for people with dementia. Many times, they couldn't get visits from their loved ones, even those who lived nearby because of the danger of infection. Organizations dedicated to fighting dementia had to work harder than ever to help people with dementia to keep their dignity and remain social through all available means.

But the pandemic isn't the only enemy of dementia socialization. There's a lot of prejudice associated with dementia, and many people step back when someone is diagnosed with it. Even close friends and family members feel they are wasting their time dealing with a dementia patient, and can't deal with the frustration and repetition of dealing with them. Instead of adapting, they step away, which has a devastating impact on the patient's health.

As the caregiver, you can plan many activities that you and your loved one can do together, and with the presence of others. That could be as simple as getting people together to listen to calming music, playing a board game, tending to a garden, or having a pleasant conversation. Find out what they would like to do and keep doing it. This will keep them happy and benefit their mind and spirit.

If you can't dedicate your entire day to your loved one, try to find an adult daycare where you can leave your loved one for a few hours. These are places dedicated to patients with dementia, and have a staff dedicated to treat this kind of patient, while promoting socialization and taking care of your loved one's hygiene. Unlike a nursing home, this is a place where older adults stay for a limited time each day while their caregivers go to work and take care of their chores, like at a children's daycare.

Faith can have a powerful effect on making people feel like they belong to a community. Don't force faith into your loved one's life if they weren't religious before dementia, or if they were from a different faith than you profess. The most important thing is the activities and people that are involved in this environment, the feeling of belonging, and the sensation of doing something meaningful.

Early diagnosis is crucial in dementia, and Wetherell and Jeste (2003) have created the method known as Decision Tree for Early Detection of Cognitive Impairment by Community Pharmacists, which works by asking the following questions:

- Is there impairment in memory plus one of the following: aphasia, apraxia, agnosia, disturbance in executive functioning?
- Does it interfere with their social skills?
- Does it differentiate from delirium, depression, intoxication, mental retardation, psychopathology, malingering?
- Does the patient have dementia alone or dementia with some other comorbid condition, such as delirium, depression, substance abuse, or medical conditions? Is there any head trauma, substance abuse, or anoxia as contributing factors?
- What is the history of the patient's dementia?

 Sometimes, it takes more courage to ask for help than to act alone.

— KEN PETTI

You should never allow yourself to lose your courage during your journey as a caregiver. You need help, and so does your loved one or patient. Seek it, build it, and enforce it with a visual aid. Once they can't take care of themselves anymore, it may be time for you to get your home ready.

GETTING YOUR HOME READY FOR WHEN THEY CAN'T LIVE ALONE

a regular house environment offers many hazards to a dementia patient. Don't wait until the later stages of dementia to make the necessary modifications in that environment to prevent accidents and make sure that your loved one can perform their daily activities. At some point, they will no longer be able to live alone, but until then they should be able to get everything they need without the risk of falling, burning themselves, or suffering any other accident.

It's also important that the dementia patient is unable to hurt themselves. According to De Jonghe-Rouleau *et al.* (2005b), 22% of dementia patients adopt self-harm behaviors, by scratching themselves or banging their fists against objects. While you can't fully control that self-destructive behavior, it's still your job to make it difficult for them to do so.

WHEN THEY CAN NO LONGER LIVE BY THEMSELVES

Dementia is a progressive condition, and even though its first signs are mild, they get worse overtime. The symptoms grow and change, making it difficult for a person to conduct their daily activities to the point they need constant care. By then, they can't live independently any longer, and will need a caregiver.

Each case of dementia is unique, and there's no specific rule for determining whether someone needs full-time care. The family should watch them closely, consult with their doctor, and make a decision based on several factors. Based on how fast it progresses and the symptoms they're experiencing, not every family can provide the treatment and care that a dementia patient needs.

Depending on the type of dementia and how far into it they are, the dementia patient should have a voice in the decision. However, there are cases in which they can't advocate for their own self-interest. They may feel there's nothing wrong with them, while having problems with hygiene, organization, feeding, communication, movement, and their general well-being.

Some families choose part-time care, having someone pay regular visits to the dementia patient, preparing their meals, cleaning the house, and shopping for groceries. With time that may not be enough, and the solution is to opt for a full-time professional who can assist the dementia patient with their chores.

Choosing full-time care shouldn't feel like a defeat, though it often does, with families refusing to accept that their loved one can't take care of themselves anymore. With time it becomes hard to ignore the signs, such as a foul body odor that shows a lack of hygiene, strange weight loss, or a messy house.

It's not easy for someone who is used to having independence having someone assisting them at all times. But full-time care isn't just about watching over a senior person to keep them from falling. It's about restoring their dignity through companionship. Dementia causes isolation and confusion, and the caregiver's job is to help them to re-socialize and find joy in small things.

ADAPTING YOUR HOUSE

Self-harm is a serious problem for people with dementia. You'd be amazed by how many disastrous scenarios could happen in a simple environment, such as a kitchen or a bathroom. You want to make sure that your loved one isn't in danger during day-to-day situations, like having a meal or walking around the house.

Securing the Kitchen

A normal home kitchen is one of the most accident-prone rooms in any house. You can remove a lot of risks with sturdy furniture and removing rugs completely. The kitchen should be well-lit so you can observe your loved one having their meals. Make sure that the chairs are ergonomic and easy to get in and out if you have to attend to an emergency. Chairs should also be well padded, not only for comfort, but to make sure their legs don't fall asleep. Avoid getting pedestal tables and give preference to heavy tables that feel sturdy when you touch them. All of this will come in handy in an emergency, such as your loved one choking on their food.

Wet floors are the major cause of falls in the kitchen. You should apply a non-slippery coat or a non-skid adhesive on the floor, especially if it's made of tiles as the area around the sink gets wet. If your loved one is using a walker, consider getting them a special tray trolley, which includes a surface where they can rest plates and cups. Also remove all rugs and mats, especially if they're worn out.

Once you have safe furniture, it's time to take care of the kitchen appliances. Stoves are the most dangerous ones, with gas stoves being the worst. The dementia patient may wake up in the middle of the night and decide to use the stove or the oven, which could lead to gas leaking or burns. To avoid that, remove the oven knobs and turn the gas off when you're not using it. You can also buy special locks for that purpose. Attaching an isolation valve to a gas cooker will shut it off if the gas keeps leaking while unlit.

Electric kettles are safer than stove-top kettles as they have an automatic switch that turns it off once the water has boiled. That saves energy and also decreases the risk of a short-circuit. A dementia patient may still scald themselves while operating one of these, especially if they overfill it, so it's better to always have someone to assist them.

Blending colors makes a difference for a dementia patient when identifying boundaries. Get a tablecloth that contrasts with the floor, otherwise you could cause visual confusion and make them trip. Keep everything as clean as possible, making sure that sharp objects are beyond their reach, and tuck away cords on which they could trip.

Refrigerators pose a different danger. A dementia patient who has full access to the refrigerator may eat anything they find in there, including raw and old food, as well as alcoholic beverages they're not supposed to drink and food they're allergic to. There's also the danger of dropping glass jars that could cause them to cut themselves.

A dementia patient shouldn't have access to the microwave, for they won't always remember the danger of putting metal or aluminum inside of it. Other small appliances, such as blenders, food processors, coffeemakers, tea kettles, coffee grinders, and stand mixers also offer different types of danger. It's better to keep them in a locked cabinet, accessing them only when they're necessary.

Keep a fire extinguisher in the kitchen in a strategic place, and take the time to learn how to use it. You should also teach your loved one how to use the fire extinguisher, so they can be prepared in an extreme situation. Smoke detectors and carbon monoxide detectors also make a difference, but you need to make sure their batteries are charged.

Cooking is a therapeutic activity, though not the safest one for a dementia patient. If the person has cooked for themselves their entire lives, depriving them from it could have a negative effect. Still, you should watch over your loved one with dementia while they cook. Electric cookers are helpful in the kitchen, and you can use an electric cook guard to monitor their functioning. If the appliance goes too hot, the guard will sound an alarm.

When adapting your kitchen for a dementia patient, don't overlook water faucets and garbage disposals. A running faucet could flood the kitchen and a hot water tap could scald them. There are automatic shutoff devices and anti-scalding faucet controls you can install to avoid that. A dementia patient may stuff the garbage disposal and, at worse, stick their hand in there and get injured. While some garbage disposals only work with a running faucet, there are also models that only run if they have a cover in place.

Cabinets and cupboards hold many dangers to seniors with dementia. Pots and pans, as well as dishes, glasses, and other breakable items may fall on their heads. They may also be able to access knives, cleaning products, plastic bags, spices, and many other hazardous things they might mistake for food. Installing simple child-proof safety latches will save you a lot of headaches.

People with hand tremors can benefit from heavier utensils, which you can find in regular cookware stores. A dementia patient needs to have some items within reach. You don't want them to climb up onto the cupboard to get a bottle opener or a Tupperware lid, and it's better to have plenty of those around the house. Your loved one may also get attached to a mug or a cup. If so, make sure it's heavy-duty and non-breakable.

People with dementia have a tendency of mistaking objects for food, especially artificial fruit and refrigerator magnets in the shape of food. Get rid of those, and any other object that looks delicious but isn't. If you're keeping a real fruit basket, make sure the fruit is fresh and that your loved one isn't allergic to it. Also avoid flower arrangements in the kitchen, artificial or not.

Considering that even people without dementia get sick from eating expired food, it's important to keep an eye out for them. Rotting food can also cause roaches and other vermin. Keep notes on the fridge door specifying when something needs to be thrown out.

Securing the Bathroom

With slippery floors, increased humidity, and obstacles such as rugs, toilets, and bidets, the bathroom is one of the most dangerous places in the house for a dementia patient. It's important that the bathroom is well-lilt and clean to avoid cockroaches and other vermin. Apart from asking a nurse to pay a visit to your home and evaluate the conditions of your bathroom, there are some modifications that you can perform yourself.

One of the most essential items is a shower chair, in which the dementia patient can sit while taking a shower or a bath. You'll find that sitting baths are more comfortable for you and the person you're taking care of. Non-skid strips are ideal to avoid slipping and falling, and you should also install grab bars which they can use for support while bathing or using the toilet.

People have their preferences regarding baths or showers, but that can change as a person develops dementia. Talk to your loved one about what they're most comfortable with, and adapt your bathroom accordingly. Make the bathing process fun, encouraging your loved one to take part instead of doing all the work yourself. Make sure you clean the most sensitive areas, such the genitals, buttocks, and perineum, even if that feels awkward.

There's always a danger that people with dementia will lock themselves inside rooms, but that's worse with bathrooms. You need to remove the locks from the bathroom door, and you should always accompany your loved one into the bathroom when they're using it. Apart from preventing accidents, you also need to guarantee they're cleaning themselves properly after using the toilet.

When choosing items such as soap, toothbrushes, and face towels, pick those with vibrant colors. That will keep the bathroom visually interesting and make it easier for everyone to identify different objects with no effort. For the same reason, the toilet seat color should contrast with the bowl. If the bathroom is connected to the person's bedroom, you can install a motion sensor that will tell you when they're using it.

Faucets may look harmless, but they can hurt your loved one if they hit its tip. The same foam or rubber faucet covers that are used for small children are helpful for senior people. Having the hot and cold water coming from the same faucet allows you to mix temperatures and avoid burns.

Electrical appliances are a danger in the bathroom, because of the constant presence of water. You can use GFI or plastic socket inserts or covers to prevent electrical shock. Another risk is to have prescription and nonprescription medication stored in the bathroom cabinet. Instead, keep those in a locked cabinet.

Securing the Bedroom

Even if you're going to sleep in the same bedroom as the dementia patient, it's hard to monitor them during the entire night. People leave the bedroom for different reasons in the middle of the night, and you can't risk having your loved one wandering around the house while you sleep. The most basic thing you can do is to meet their night needs, so they won't get out of bed to use the bathroom or have a snack or a glass of water.

That doesn't cover all contingencies, and you might have to invest in a motion sensor to wake you up whenever your loved one gets out of bed during the night. If you're sleeping in different rooms, you'll also need a monitoring device that will alert you if the person falls from the bed.

Scatter rugs and throw rugs are a danger for people with dementia, but mats can make a difference between a bruise and a broken bone if you place them strategically around the bed. During the cold season, avoid electric blankets and heating pads, which can burn your loved one. During warmer weather, get secure portable fans that can't get jammed with objects between their blades.

Securing Other Areas

When taking care of a dementia patient, common features of your house may turn into a recipe for disaster. Electrical cords around the living room can cause people to fall, glass doors can become invisible obstacles, and fireplaces become a liability. There are simple solutions to these issues, such as rubber organizers for the cords, stickers for the glass doors, and alternative sources of heat.

A common laundry room is filled with chemical products that can cause serious harm if ingested. Because of that, you should always keep the laundry door locked, and, to be extra safe, keep these products in a locked cabinet. Don't let the dementia patient operate the laundry machinery, especially electric irons.

The dementia patient shouldn't have access to basements, sheds, garages, or any place in which you store tools, machines, and vehicles. Even simple sporting equipment could become a weapon for them to hurt themselves or other people. They may also feel the urge to use a vehicle to escape home. Even if they can't operate the vehicle, this can be dangerous.

Fire Protection

Investing in a good smoke alarm system and carbon monoxide detectors can save lives. Instead of buying and installing one by yourself, hire a professional to come to your house. Not only will they perform a proper installation, but they will also explain how the device works and all the important procedures.

Hallways and the top of stairs are the ideal places to install smoke alarms. Placing them in kitchens and bathrooms could unnecessarily set them off as they are sensitive to changes in temperature. They are powered by batteries, and you should check them periodically to make sure they have enough power.

Door Alarms

One of the scariest scenarios for a caregiver is the discovery that their loved one has walked out of the house. You can avoid that by making your front door more secure with extra latches, but a door alarm is a more reliable solution. These devices tell you when someone is entering or leaving the house, or when they're walking around between different rooms.

Taking Them Outside

You may feel tempted to keep your loved one inside the house, where everything is controlled. However, taking them outside will relieve stress and strengthen your bonds. The same principles from inside the house apply here—eliminating objects where they may trip, installing non-skid strips in slippery surfaces, having bars for them to hold on to, etc.

Gardening can be a pleasant activity for a dementia patient, but you need to follow their movements, so they won't hurt themselves with gardening tools and dangerous plants. If you have a swimming pool, keep it covered at all times, and only let them use it under supervision. A motion sensor that turns lights on automatically will keep them from walking in the dark.

CHAPTER 5 PRACTICAL EXERCISE

Here's a checklist of all the steps we've seen in this chapter. Mark the ones you've already met, and attempt to meet the other ones.

Kitchen

- lighting
- sturdy furniture
- safe rugs with rubber bottoms
- ergonomic and well-padded chairs
- non-slippery coat or a non-skid adhesive on the floor
- special tray trolley
- remove all rugs and mats
- remove the oven's knobs

- isolation valve to a gas cooker
- electric kettles
- tablecloth that contrasts with the floor
- tuck away chords
- lock refrigerators
- keep microwaves in a locked cabinet
- keep a fire extinguisher in the kitchen
- anti-scalding faucets and covered garbage disposals
- get rid of objects that may look like food

Bathroom

- shower chair
- handlebars
- non-skid strips
- remove locks from doors
- get items with vibrant colors
- foam or rubber faucet covers
- avoid electrical equipment in the bathroom
- keep medicines locked

Bedroom

- motion sensors
- mats around the bed
- avoid rugs
- avoid electric mats and blankets
- secure fans

Other areas

- stickers in glass doors
- lock the laundry
- lock the garage

Fire Protection

- smoke alarms installed by a professional
- check the batteries regularly

Door Alarms

- outside alarms to keep them from wandering
- inside alarms to know in which room they are

Taking Them Outside

- watch for gardening tools
- watch for dangerous plants and bugs

 It is not how much you do, but how much love you put into doing.

— MOTHER TERESA

The day you move your loved one to a new environment will be a challenge. Being in control of their environment will make you feel more secure. Nobody can be in control at all times, but with discipline and consistency, you can create a better environment for you and your loved ones. If you're moving them into your home, then it's time to start working on communication skills because they're likely progressing through their disease. That's what we'll see in the next chapter.

6

DISCOVERING A NEW FORM OF COMMUNICATION WITH DEMENTIA

*C*ommunicating with someone who has dementia can be challenging. It will require you to develop a new way of understanding and being understood. People with dementia can't always convey messages or express their needs. Things will be tough but it's all a matter of being open to learning new things.

For each dementia patient, there are new cues that you need to learn. Sometimes, they will call people and objects by the wrong name. In others, they will struggle to remember the name of something. That confusion generates frustration and stress, and your job is to help them remember them without losing patience.

The middle stage of dementia can last for several years, and it's important to establish early on your new ways of communicating. Instead of insisting that your loved one remember things and forcing them to call them by their right name, you need to be flexible and accept this new way of speaking. That will help you connect with that person's mind, to comprehend how their mind works, what has been lost, and what remains and can be saved.

WHAT CAN YOU EXPECT?

There will always be variations regarding how much memory each person loses through dementia. As stated, they might call things by improper names, have difficulty finding the right words, and repeat familiar words constantly. You'll often catch them losing their train of thought in the middle of a sentence as they try to organize the words in their mind with little success.

All of this generates frustration that leads the dementia patient to speak less often. People whose mother tongue isn't English will resort to their native language as a way of expressing themselves, and use hand gestures to express something they can't convey with words.

While it's important to be aware and be respectful about the speaking abilities of your loved one, you shouldn't exclude them from conversations or assume that they are having difficulties when they're not. Listen to what they have to say and take their words into account, without interrupting or trying to complete the phrase for them. They might need more time to express themselves, and you should give them that time. Also, don't ask the patient "Do you remember when x,y,z happened?" (results in frustration) but rather say "I remember when x,y,z happened" and note if it triggers a favorable reaction and then continue with the story.

COMMUNICATION IN THE MILDER STAGES OF DEMENTIA

People with dementia may feel better communicating at a specific time of the day, if possible in a pleasant, well-lit, and uncrowded environment. They might also communicate better when they are clean and well fed.

You shouldn't treat the dementia patient like a child or talk down to them. Keep eye contact, speaking at a reasonable pace with short sentences, and let them have the time they need to respond. It's important that they speak as much as they need, instead of just listening to you. They may repeat phrases and ideas, and you have to acknowledge it each time and encourage them to keep going.

If you interrupt the dementia patient, they will feel what they're saying isn't important. The same will happen if you're busy with another activity during the conversation. Cut off all distractions such as radio and TV, so you can pay attention to their verbal and nonverbal cues.

You can also use visual cues, gesturing and pointing at things to make the conversation more dynamic. Offer them choices, such as bringing a tray with orange and apple juice and asking them which one they prefer. This is a game of patience, and if you criticize, argue, or correct them too much, it will make it difficult for you to engage in a conversation again.

COMMUNICATION IN THE MIDDLE STAGES OF DEMENTIA

Engaging in a conversation gets more frustrating as dementia continues to develop. Start easy with shorter conversations, and let them express themselves. If you have other people around, try to include the dementia patient in the conversation instead of having them sitting quietly in the corner. Discuss subjects that interested them in the past, always using a friendly tone and using basic words.

At this stage the patient starts forgetting people around them. Resist the temptation to refer to them as family members, and instead introduce yourself by your first name. When they speak, you need to listen, and not just pretend to listen. You also need to observe their faces and gestures to find the cues to continue the conversation, even if what they say doesn't make sense.

It's common for people with dementia to have difficulty finding words to express themselves. Instead of providing them with the words, try to guide them until they find the words. Nodding, smiling, and saying yes or no from time to time will reassure them that you are paying attention. You need to enter their world, understand their frustrations, give them time to think and respond, and let them express what they're feeling.

Objects near you can become good prompts for conversation. You can ask them where they got a decorative item, or use that same piece to represent something else while making a point. Your loved one may start to mix different events and people in their head, and there's no point in correcting them. Stick to the main idea and let them carry on the conversation.

People with dementia still have a sense of humor, and you can have fun with jokes and games. Your loved one shouldn't feel that you are laughing at them, but with them. You may feel they're too fixed in a topic, but it's their choice whether to change the subject.

COMMUNICATION IN THE LATE STAGES OF DEMENTIA

The rules are different in the late stages of dementia. If you haven't been taking care of yourself, start as soon as possible. These conversations can be long and frustrating, and leave you exhausted.

Once again it's better to find a calm place without noise or distractions. Speak with a friendly tone, using simple words and ideas, delivered in complete sentences. Gestures and body language cues are also important here. If you're asking them if they're thirsty, for example, you can mimic a gesture of drinking a glass of water.

By now the dementia patient may not remember who you and other people are, but you should always refer to everyone by their names. They have a hard time processing much information, so keep the conversation to one simple topic. If they have to make a decision, offer clear options for them to choose. For example, hold two packs of soup in front of them and ask which they prefer—chicken or tomato?

During moments of distress, people with dementia may find comfort in perfume, the texture of a teddy bear, or from you singing a specific song. Take advantage of that during your conversations. As the disease progresses, communication becomes less about two people discussing a point, and more about you trying to reach the core of your loved one and give them some peace in their daily lives.

Here are some things you should never say to a dementia patient:

- How come you don't recognize me? We've known each other for years!
- What do you do during the day?
- I've already answered that a million times!
- Don't you remember your sister died five years ago?
- Do you know what you're doing, sweetheart?
- Remember when we saw that movie?

Bringing your spouse, partner, children, or anyone at home on board the communication train will help practice these communication skills. Don't allow friends, family, or anyone else to dismiss the rules for effective communication with dementia patients. Even worse, don't let anyone, even kids, disrespect the person or make them feel undignified. Your loved one's mental health is fragile enough. Their struggle with speech, understanding, and communication can make it worse if anyone crosses the lines in this chapter. Please educate your friends and family to ensure they treat the person with respect, patience, and dignity.

CHAPTER 6 PRACTICAL EXERCISE

Print these nine rules and keep them at a visible place where you can always consult them:

1. Conduct conversations in calm and quiet places.
2. Talk in short and concise sentences.
3. Use gestures and body language to communicate with the dementia patient.
4. Use visual cues to illustrate your speech.
5. Offer options for the dementia patient to choose between.
6. Always refer to each person by their first name.
7. Don't correct the dementia patient if their ideas don't make sense.
8. Include the dementia patient in conversations that involve other people.
9. Educate your family and friends, including children, about the importance of these rules.

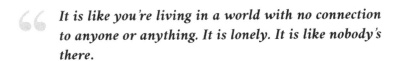

> *It is like you're living in a world with no connection to anyone or anything. It is lonely. It is like nobody's there.*

— TAMSIN CALIDAS

As you keep talking to your loved one, you'll get a sense of what it's like to be in their shoes. Losing your connection to people must be terrifying, so understand your loved one's emotional state. Next, let's focus on common medical issues and how you can address them, including mental health.

COMMON MEDICAL ISSUES AND HOW TO ADDRESS THEM

*Y*our loved one will face some medical and mental health problems. Falls and injuries are the most common type of medical emergency with older individuals, but there are many other health issues that come with age. Knowing what to expect and what to do can save their lives. It's also important to find a physician or geriatric care manager that you can rely on.

Some professionals will visit your loved one at their house and offer assistance there, but in most cases you will have to commute to their office or clinic. In other cases, only a hospital has the facilities, equipment, and professionals to heal your loved one. My mother had a visiting doctor who only charged $15 per visit as co-pay. Of course, Medicare paid the lion's share. Nobody enjoys this kind of situation, but there are some preparations that you can make in advance to make these moments less traumatic.

FEVER

Fever is characterized by having a temperature two degrees or more above one's normal temperature. It can be caused by infection, dehydration, constipation, or heat stroke. Use a digital thermometer to identify cases of fever—they're safer and more reliable than the ones made of glass.

FLU OR PNEUMONIA

Symptoms of flu and pneumonia include aches, chills, coughing, vomiting, difficulty in breathing, and dizziness. Fever is a common symptom, although it doesn't always happen in pneumonia cases. These symptoms sometimes go away and come back, and can affect other areas of a person's health.

Flu and pneumonia shots decrease the chances of seniors contracting these diseases. Citizens who are 65 or above should get their yearly flu shot. The formula is updated every year based on the scientist's predictions of how the virus is going to develop.

People suffering from the flu and pneumonia are advised to stay home to avoid spreading the illness, drink plenty of fluids, eat healthy food, and get as much rest as they can. People with dementia often depend on the visits of family and friends, and professionals such as physical therapists. If any of these people are experiencing flu symptoms, they're advised to suspend those visits until they're well.

FALLS

The dementia patient will experience trouble keeping their balance, and may have difficulty perceiving distances, which makes them prone to falls. You can avoid the chances of a fall by removing clutter and rugs, and installing grab bars.

If your loved one falls, their doctor should conduct an examination, including blood pressure and blood tests, to make sure if the patient isn't developing a new condition. It may be a serious disease, or something less threatening, like an aching foot. Doctors also need to consider the medication the patient is taking to make sure it isn't interfering with the patient's sense of balance.

DEHYDRATION

Dizziness, rapid heart rate, dry mouth, and hallucinations are symptoms of dehydration, which happens when the water level in your body is below the necessary level you need to function. A good way of making sure your loved one is getting enough fluid is by marking the hours in which they need to drink water, even if they are not thirsty.

If you suspect they are dehydrated, it's important to consult a nurse or doctor as soon as possible. In extreme cases, the patient may be unable to consume liquids, which is worse in cases of vomiting or diarrhea.

CONSTIPATION

Getting enough liquid every day is especially important to avoid constipation in senior citizens. Subtle changes in an older person's routine can mess with their system, so keep an eye on their diet, making sure they're getting enough fiber from fruits like raisins and prunes, as well as juice, gelatin, cereal, and decaffeinated coffee.

DIARRHEA

Diarrhea is a side effect of several medications, including those related to dementia. It can also be caused by other medical problems or be related to the patient's diet. Make sure your loved one is washing their hands properly after using the toilet to avoid contamination, and be extra careful with what they consume—even tap water can be dangerous. Seek medical help at the first sign of diarrhea and present the patient's entire history, including recent events, in order to arrive at a diagnosis.

INCONTINENCE

People with incontinence have no control over their bladder, which can result in awkward situations. It's a common issue with senior citizens, and can be caused by a number of reasons, from consuming too much liquid to consuming too little, diabetes, an enlarged prostate gland, urinary tract infections, or medication that makes it harder to hold urine.

You can ease the effects of incontinence by taking the person to the bathroom at regular intervals as well as whenever they feel the need. Comfortable clothes won't constrict their bladder, and are easy to remove if they do get it wet. To avoid bedwetting, limit fluids after 6 p.m., offering a piece of fruit if they're too thirsty. In some cases, you might have to invest in geriatric diapers, disposable underwear, and waterproof bed sheets.

VISION PROBLEMS

Diminishing eyesight in dementia patients may be caused by specific conditions, but can also be a side effect of some other disease, and also a result of natural aging. It can be hard to distinguish the symptoms of vision loss with those of dementia.

As dementia patients have trouble interacting with the world around them, one might consider whether that's caused by the loss of brain cells or by poor vision.

A person who has both of those conditions will be more disoriented and suffer a higher risk of falling. When taking care of a dementia patient, it's important to schedule regular appointments with an eye doctor, who may recommend glasses or eye surgery. Keeping the house environment well-lit and with plenty of contrasting colors will help them to move around.

HEARING PROBLEMS

Like with visual problems, hearing loss can also be confused with the symptoms of dementia. Hearing loss can have several causes related to noise damage, but it can be a normal part of aging. People of all ages can develop deafness, not just the older population, though there is a still not-explained connection between deafness and dementia (Sight and Hearing Loss With Dementia, n.d.).

Since dementia diagnosis depends on interviews with the patient, hearing loss makes the diagnosis more difficult. Take your loved one to regular hearing checks with a doctor. You can help them preserve what hearing they still have left with hearing aids. At the same time, you can use other forms of communication, such as gestures, lip reading, and visual clues.

DENTAL PROBLEMS

If you don't pay attention to the dementia patient's oral health, they might develop decayed teeth, sores, and lumps. They are not always able to tell you what they're feeling, and you need to pay attention to signs such as a sore mouth and bad breath.

Brushing and flossing their teeth controls dental plaque and germs, which can lead to oral diseases.

Oral cancer is a risk in older people. If you notice your loved one has trouble chewing or swallowing, and there are spots or lumps in their mouth, lips or throat, or there is a white or red patch in their mouth, take them to the dentist for exams.

PAIN

Conditions such as constipation, pressure sores, skin tears, leg ulcers, osteoarthritis, muscle rigidity, and stiffening of joints are the most common causes of pain in dementia patients. It's also related to several common diseases, such as arthritis and ulcers.

You may also find they also experience pain as they're forced to move, to go to bed or take a bath, for example. If you are unsure what's causing the pain, just ask. People in different stages of dementia are still able to communicate what's wrong with them. You can also identify at which moments they complain of pain the most, and use that to pinpoint the cause of the pain. Bring that information to the doctor on your next appointment. They might prescribe painkillers, but in some cases a simple change of routine can solve the problem.

SKINCARE, BEDSORES, AND RASHES

Age changes a person's skin, making it thinner and less smooth, as well as more sensitive to bruises and cuts, developing spots, dryness, and in some cases, cancer. You can use simple store bought lotions, moisturizers, and soaps to take care of problems like dry skin and sores. Keep your loved one's nails short so to avoid them scratching themselves.

Without the protective fatty layer, aging people bruise easily. If bruises continue to appear, it's a good idea to take them to the doctor. Pay attention to their body fold areas, such as the neck and armpits, which can get irritated and create skin tags.

Don't treat skin issues as merely cosmetic for they will interfere with your loved one's health. This becomes more serious in people who are bedridden, who need to be turned and cleaned to preserve their skin health.

MEDICATION

Dementia patients are not always willing to take their medicine. Being forced to take pills at specific times of day can be frightening, and give them the feeling that they're not in control of their own lives. Medication hour should never be distressing, and you need to provide a calm and relaxing environment at that time.

Don't overmedicate your loved one and pay attention to any side effects. If your loved one is rejecting a pill, it could be because it's actually causing them grief. Big pills can get stuck in their throat, but talk to your doctor before crushing them in smaller chunks, for not all pills are designed to be crushed.

There's no point in trying to explain the purpose of the medication, as the dementia patient can't always process that information. If they downright refuse to take the pill, walk out of the room and come back in 10 minutes to try again.

DIZZINESS, FAINTING, IMBALANCE, AND LOSS OF COORDINATION

Syncope, which is the name of dizziness that causes fainting, is a common symptom of Lewy Body dementia and other kinds of dementia. It happens when the heart rate or blood pressure drop, or when certain parts of the body don't get the necessary amount of blood. Dizziness can also be caused by some types of medicine, especially the ones related to memory, psychosis, anxiety, insomnia, and depression.

If your loved one is experiencing constant episodes of dizziness, you should invest in fall sensors, which go in their wrist and can inform you whenever they have the risk of falling. There are also special padded suits which can protect them when falling is inevitable, and instruments such as Hop'Safe, an airbag that goes around their hips and inflates to protect them.

SEIZURES

The damage that dementia causes in a person's brain can lead to seizures. Seizures are a common early sign of degenerative diseases, such as Parkinson's and Alzheimer's. Doctors can diagnose these diseases in their early stages as the causes of those seizures, which is treatable with the same kind of drugs used for epilepsy.

HOSPITAL TRIPS

You can reduce much of the stress of a hospital trip by being prepared for emergencies. Knowing which hospital to go to and having everything prepared in advance will spare them from distress. Be ready to inform the doctors of your loved one's medical history, including the medication they're taking. Don't forget to explain their stage of dementia and other illnesses they might have.

Patience is important, and you need to remain calm to be able to comfort your loved one. This situation could last for hours while you wait for lab exams. You shouldn't have to face this on your own, so don't be afraid to request the presence of a friend or family member. If the patient has to stay overnight, you might consider going back home to get some sleep, but always leave someone there with them.

You know the patient better than the doctors, and you can tell if they're behaving differently or if there's something wrong. Keep in mind that this situation is distressing for them, being in an unfamiliar environment with new medication, tests, and strange people. They need your emotional assistance as much as everything else.

CHAPTER 7 PRACTICAL EXERCISE

Here's a bullet list of what your loved one may be suffering from. Don't forget to take all of these into consideration whenever they assume an unusual behavior.

- fever
- flu
- pneumonia
- falls
- dehydration
- constipation
- diarrhea
- incontinence
- vision problems
- hearing problems
- dental problems
- pain
- bedsores, and rashes
- dizziness
- fainting
- imbalance
- loss of coordination
- seizures

You gain strength, courage, and confidence by every experience in which you really stop to look fear in the face. You must do the things which you think you cannot do.

— ELEANOR ROOSEVELT

At times you may feel powerless and wonder if you're doing a good job as a caregiver. Never doubt how you can help your loved one or patient at home, even when you're alone. You now know when and how to seek help. So, let's look at daily struggles and how to address each.

8

PRACTICAL EVERYDAY CARE FOR
A LOVED ONE WITH DEMENTIA

$\mathcal{A}$s your loved one's dementia worsens, some daily challenges will arise. They will have trouble fulfilling their ADLs such as bathing, eating, and dressing. At first you may feel uncomfortable assisting in wiping your loved one after they use the toilet or giving them a bath, but it's crucial that you overcome that barrier, for personal hygiene is crucial for their health.

There are some actions you can take to make bath time less intrusive for you and the person you're taking care of. They might fight you if you try to undress them and lead them to the shower or bathtub. Once again patience is key, and it also helps to make the bath a pleasant and relaxing experience. Use warm water and find out what kind of soap and shampoo your loved one enjoys the most. All of that will help them to accept this new reality, and with time they will accept it as a natural part of their daily lives.

HYGIENE

Lack of hygiene is a serious problem for dementia patients, and if you don't monitor it, it can lead to serious health issues. Imagine how discomforting it feels to have another person assisting you while doing private activities such as bathing and shaving. You'll need their collaboration in this, and a friendly approach gives the best results.

Establish a routine for bathing, choosing the time of the day when your loved one is relaxed. You can bathe, shower, or sponge bath them based on their own preference. Let them feel the temperature of the water and adjust it until they like it. Some dementia patients are afraid of the water, due to its depth or temperature. Don't force them to confront that fear, and instead offer them options.

Bathing time and hair washing time should be kept separate for patients with long hair. If you feel your loved one is getting too agitated at hair washing time, consider taking them to a hair-dresser. You can also ask the hairdresser to come to the home to wash and cut your loved one's hair in a familiar environment.

Another potentially discomforting moment is toileting. They may not be ready to have an assistant at such a personal moment, but it's risky to let them handle it by themselves— which becomes more serious when they're suffering from incontinence. Make sure they are clean and change their under-wear if needed. They might need a complete change of clothes, and there should always be clean ones available for this kind of situation.

At the first stages of dementia, patients may still be allowed to shave by themselves, and all you have to do is remind them. As dementia progresses, you can get them an electric razor, which offers less risks, or you can shave them yourself. You also need to remind them to clean their ears, for an excessive amount of earwax can damage their hearing. Cutting fingernails will prevent them from hurting themselves.

NUTRITION

Some eating problems are caused by old age, but people with dementia may also forget when to eat and drink, how to cook, and use utensils. Their medication may also affect their appetite, and they have trouble communicating when they're hungry or full. You have to pay close attention to your loved one during mealtimes, limit distractions at the table, and give them plenty of time to finish their meal.

Allow the dementia patient to be independent as they eat, using their abilities of handling food and instruments. A good alternative is serving finger foods, with bite-sized portions that they can handle with their hands. They might make a mess at the table, but you can always clean it later. Avoid foods that are hard to chew or swallow or foods with strange appearance that the patient may not recognize.

Your loved one may become agitated if their food is too hot or cold, if the place is too crowded or noisy, or if you give them too much assistance. They can also get frustrated if the food is too bland. Spices, herbs, and gravies are the best solution to make these more appetizing—just beware not to make it too spicy.

If you notice your loved one is having trouble chewing or swallowing, you can offer moist foods or liquid dietary supplements, which should be prescribed by a doctor. These supplements can also be served between meals. Remember that the patient should be fed during specific meal times, and not when they complain that they are hungry—people with severe dementia often forget how to eat.

A balanced diet should be rich in:

- protein (fish, meat, eggs, nuts, beans)
- fruits and vegetables
- oils
- dairy
- grains

You should also avoid fried foods with high saturated fat and cholesterol, and reduce the consumption of sugar and salt.

EXERCISE AND PHYSICAL ACTIVITY

Like any other person, dementia patients can benefit from regular exercise. Though not a cure for dementia, exercise can help the patient strengthen their bodies, stay at a healthy weight, and keep them in a better mood. Cardiovascular workouts bring the most benefits, but they should also be monitored to avoid incidents during the workout due to their inherent problems with balance and visual perception. Those can lead to falls or injuries with the workout instruments.

People who are older won't be able to work out at the same rate as younger persons. Their coordination and endurance aren't as strong, and they may have sore feet and muscles as well as the many illnesses that come with old age. If your loved one can't take long walks or go to the gym, they can still use a stationary bike, stretching bands, and lift weights. Don't encourage them to do more than is reasonable, which could harm them.

Each person may enjoy working out much more at specific hours. Learn which ones suit your loved one best. They may feel better taking a walk in the morning instead of the evening. Find a pleasant place for that walk, if possible one where other people take their walk at the same time—even better if some of those people are the same age as your loved one!

RECREATION

An active mind will better resist the decline caused by dementia. Recreational activities can train the brain like a muscle, making it stronger against issues such as memory loss. A dementia patient should enjoy plenty of outdoor activity to keep their minds happy and occupied, but it's also possible to find joy indoors playing board games solving puzzle blocks or crosswords. Another great way of taking care of one's mind is to look at old pictures and talk about the images with the rest of the family.

The idea of an older person playing video games or learning a musical instrument may seem strange, but this kind of activity can be rewarding. A dementia patient who speaks more than one language can benefit from having conversations in those languages. All of this will help reduce the amount of brain cell damage and may keep brain cells from dying.

SLEEP ISSUES

This is a serious issue for people with mild to moderate dementia, and it gets even worse during the severe stages. It causes people to be sleepy during the day and have insomnia at night— whether it's having trouble falling asleep, waking up in the middle of the night, or having premature morning awakenings.

Insomnia and other sleeping issues can be caused by exhaustion, confusion, stress, frustration, or a disruption in the internal body clock. That happens when the person doesn't establish a routine for going to bed and waking up. Bad dreams and a stressful environment also make it hard for one to fall and remain asleep.

Insomnia can be a symptom for underlying conditions, such as sleep apnea or depression. It can also be caused by the lack of physical activity, consumption of stimulants such as alcohol and caffeine, and too much screen time before going to bed. It can also happen when one takes or stops taking a specific medication.

Be gentle with your loved one when they wake up in the middle of the night, and try to assess what's wrong with them. It can be as simple as getting them another blanket or taking them to the toilet. If they ask to turn on the TV or to get dressed, explain to them that it's nighttime, and that they need to go back to bed.

Some doctors will prescribe sleep-inducing medications. This kind of medication increases the risk of falls and confusion in older people, which can cause more problems than it solves.

As the caregiver, you also need to get enough sleep to be able to take care of your loved one with dementia. You may feel tempted to use nighttime to do things you couldn't do when your loved one is awake, but that is precious sleeping time that you're missing, and it will have an impact on your daytime behavior.

CHAPTER 8 PRACTICAL EXERCISE

Here are some strategies that you can use to establish a routine of activities in your daily life:

1. Instead of creating a routine from scratch, use what you already have. Does the person with dementia like to have a specific breakfast? Do they have a favorite TV

show? Do they like to take their bath before going to bed? Adapt your own ideas to this pre-existing routine, and that will make things easier.

2. Be ready for changes in that routine as dementia progresses. If your loved one decides they don't like to watch football games on the TV anymore, you might suggest a movie, or you could play a game together.

3. Get your loved one involved in the house routine, even if they can't assist you. You can put a chair in a place where they can watch you do the laundry as you have a conversation, or bring them to the garden to help you prune the plants.

4. Making physical exercise part of a routine is crucial for anyone who wants to get in shape. Apply that to your loved one's daily schedule, taking them for walks or doing other forms of exercise at the same time of the day.

5. Save a portion of the day to sit down and listen to music. It could be classical music, folk songs, or anything that the dementia patient enjoys—only avoid songs that are too aggressive and/or profane.

 Worry never robs tomorrow of its sorrow; it only robs today of its joy.

— LEO BUSCAGLIA

During your journey as a caregiver, you are asked to put everything aside to take care of someone who cannot take care of themselves. This requires self-abnegation, which doesn't mean you should stop caring for yourself. Not only because you need to be in good mental and physical shape to conduct that job, but also because you are a human being with your own needs and dreams. When this journey ends, you will have to be in one piece to continue your life. That's part of what we'll see in the next chapter.

9

DON'T FORGET TO CARE FOR YOUR AND YOUR FAMILY'S WELL-BEING

$\mathcal{I}$f you don't make an effort to balance your professional and personal life with your caregiving, you won't be able to do anything right. While this is an activity that requires commitment, nobody can expect you to throw everything away and dedicate 100% to your loved one with dementia.

Over 30% of caregivers don't get enough sleep, and nearly 15% of them struggle with mental health almost every second day (Hitt, 2023). Let's see how you can avoid mental health challenges during the caregiving years.

TIME MANAGEMENT

While taking care of the needs of a loved one with dementia, people forget how to take care of themselves. It's paramount that you watch over your own mind, spirit, and body, not only for your own sake, but for the sake of the person you're looking after. There will be situations in which you need to take a deep breath and be the strongest person you can be, and the only way of doing that is by watching over yourself.

105

It's difficult to maintain your social and professional life while also being a caregiver. This can be a lonely job, and you will have to be by your loved one's side at moments you wish you could be elsewhere. But it's possible to find a compromise. It's not selfish to ask for a family member to take care of your loved one while you go out to see a movie or go on a date.

Planning ahead will help you to save some time that you can use for your own activities. A caregiver's daily activities should always be planned, and applying this to your "me time" will help you to enjoy them. If you share your tasks with other caregivers, such as your siblings, you need to establish who is going to do what at what time. This way, you don't duplicate tasks and avoid wasting precious time.

If you're going out tonight and you're leaving your loved one home with your brother, the last thing you want is to find out you're out of diapers—which were your responsibility. Someone has to stay with the person with dementia while the other goes out to buy the diapers, which will ruin all of your plans.

With time your caregiving responsibilities will increase, and your chances of free time decrease. Enjoy every chance you have to go out and meet people, trying to be mindful at the present moment and not your responsibilities back home.

Being mindful is also important when building a career at the same time you take care of your loved one. Talk to people at work and let them know about your role as a caregiver, not as a way of getting special treatment, but so they know you are committed to getting a balance between the two activities.

If you're not an organized person, prepare to change that. Living in a cluttered home can make you exhausted, and makes it much harder to do everything we've discussed so far. It's not only a matter of aesthetics—being able to find something at the right time, without looking all around the house, can be a matter of life and death.

Taking care of yourself goes beyond that, though. It involves looking for medical, psychiatric, psychological, and spiritual help for yourself. You need to stay in control of your body, eating well and exercising, and taking medication if necessary. Regular sessions with a psychologist will help you blow off some steam, and you may also find comfort in going to church and talking to other people in similar situations.

Here are some online resources that may help you:

- Family Caregiver Alliance's Online Caregiver Support Group: A mail-based system in which you can ask for and receive assistance in several topics regarding dementia.
- Caregiver Support Group: a regular session hosted by HopeHealth on Zoom, to answer the questions of dementia caregivers.
- Caregiver Nation: With over a thousand family caregiver members, this Facebook group is a safe place to share information, ask questions, or look for support.
- ALZConnected: Free online community with two forums for people with Alzheimer's and for their caretakers.
- Memory People: Facebook group with over 24,000 members where people can share their stories and look for support.
- Alzheimer's and Dementia Caregivers Support Chat Group: A Facebook group for caregivers, family members, and friends of people with dementia to share their experiences.
- Smart Patients: A huge online community of support dedicated not only to people with dementia, but other

mental and neurodegenerative disorders such as dementia.

Using these forums and resources will make you realize you don't have to be the strongest person in the world, and that other people have and continue to walk the same path as you. Don't let dementia harm your personal relationships and isolate you from the world.

SETTING LIMITS

Morrisette (2023) presents the 80-20 rule, also known as the Pareto Principle, which dictates that 20% of a person's activities results in 80% of the results they get. It's a matter of finding out what your 20% activities are and giving them priority. For example, you may figure out that the 20% of your time that you take cleaning your loved one's room will prevent all the cleanliness problems that could cause them discomfort or illness.

You may be spending more time than you need on a specific activity. If you conduct a time audit, you may find that you could optimize that activity, or eliminate it from your schedule altogether. This way, you can set time constraints and make everything go smoothly. Your loved one may love mashed potatoes, but can they taste the difference between the one that you boiled for forty minutes and mashed yourself, or will they like instant mash just as well?

When you start optimizing your time, you'll realize there's a lot you can do for yourself. Pass on that philosophy to other caregivers, teaching them the time limitations, and discussing potential solutions. Some of them may find it hard to ask for help, and you might have to reach out to them first.

Instead of having everyone doing the same thing at different times, you can delegate certain activities to be done by certain members of your caregiving circle. This way you can employ each person's strengths and resources. You might have a cousin who drives a truck that would be ideal to do the shopping. Another relative might be a great cook, and can prepare a pot of soup on the weekend for you to freeze in batches and thaw during the week.

Every caregiver is donating their time, and it would be unfair to get upset and aggressive toward them. If someone isn't doing their job right, you need to have a frank conversation and explain what needs to be improved. You shouldn't expect perfection from yourself either. Whenever you make a mistake, try to learn from it instead of torturing yourself over it.

OVERCOMING CHALLENGES

Having a supportive spouse makes a huge difference in the life of a caregiver. Still, you shouldn't expect your other half to be a stoic, selfless martyr who endures everything without complaining. They still expect you to fulfill your role as a husband or a wife, which you can't neglect.

To keep the flame alive, it's important to stay connected with your partner, sending messages and reconnecting from time to time. When you're together, talk about pleasant experiences you had together, and show your admiration for each other. Schedule a date at a nice restaurant once a week, even if that means leaving your loved one with dementia under someone else's care.

Another aspect of your life you can't ignore is your children. They need you just as much as the person with dementia, and it's not easy to juggle these different relationships. At least once a day you should take time to connect with your child and say that you love them. Teaching them how to brush their teeth, comb their hair, and tie their shoes may seem like small activities, but they will matter to them.

One of the hardest decisions that you'll have to make is to decide if your loved one needs assisted living. While most seniors prefer to stay in their home, being cared for by a relative, that can become a challenge as the dementia progresses. A specialized home that offers 24/7 care with nurses and other professionals who can take better care of dementia patients.

Caregivers often experience a decrease in their own life quality, and find they can't perform this role anymore. If that's your case, don't feel guilty. Good quality assisted living might be what your loved one has been needing. You can and should visit them at every opportunity, always checking that they've been treated well.

WHEN THE JOURNEY ENDS

After experiencing months or years of taking care of someone, grieving for them is a strange feeling. It's impossible to hide the relief of knowing that they're resting and that you will be able to continue on with your life. Acknowledge all of your feelings, good or bad, allowing yourself to cry and yell, and letting all the pain go through you.

No two people deal with grief the same way. Your process is your own, and it will be influenced by the time you spent taking care of your loved one. Don't worry if your grief lasts longer than you expected, and don't deny it.

Find someone who you can trust to talk about what you're going through. If you still don't have a therapist, now is the time to look for one. Check with your health insurance company for a list of therapists covered under your plan. There are also free support groups for grieving caregivers, where you can talk with other people going through the same process.

CHAPTER 9 PRACTICAL EXERCISE

Smith (2018) proposes a five-step exercise that can help you to control your anxiety and panic. Take a deep breath and follow the following steps.

- Be aware of FIVE things around you, any objects in the surrounding environment.
- Be aware of FOUR things around you that you can touch.
- Be aware of THREE things you can hear.
- Be aware of TWO things you can smell.
- Be aware of ONE thing you can taste.

Use this exercise in moments of anxiety and it will help you to keep your mind in the present moment, instead of entertaining anxious thoughts.

 If you find yourself caring for a relative with dementia, the chances are you'll need help.

— PHYLLIS LOGAN

You've come a long way and adopted many tools. It's time to use them. Believe in yourself, and ensure you follow each step. Combine and reinterpret them according to your needs and beliefs, always keeping in mind that you're doing something amazing for someone who needs you. That is a reward in itself.

AFTERWORD

As we arrive at the end of the book, I'd like to invite you to recall everything you've read, and reflect on what you've learned during our journey. You now know more than you did about dementia. I hope that, as you read the book, you can identify what you had been doing right and wrong, and apply that to your own actions.

There were nine chapters in this book, designed to help you take care of your loved one with dementia. Receiving the diagnosis is never easy, and knowing how to deal with that situation will make a big difference to you and the person you're taking care of. Dementia is a progressive disease, and once the diagnosis comes, you need to learn fast and adapt to that new reality.

Does all of this feel like too much? I feel for you because I've been in your shoes. The life of a caregiver is full of uncertainties, but so is life. Anyone who claims they have all the answers is just trying to deceive you to sell more books. That's not what I planned with *Compassionate Care—Navigating Dementia Together*. The major goal of this book is to connect with people who are going through this struggle, and let you know you are not alone.

The lack of support and education can be most challenging. People have their own life to live, and some may feel that caring for a dementia patient will slow them down. Dementia may erase a person's memory, but it doesn't erase the past. Old pains and grudges may still get in the way for some people.

It took me time and patience to gain the information I've shared here with you. If I could ask for one thing in return is for you to share what you discovered today. Leave a comment or review to help others find this information. Beyond that, I wish you all the best and many joyous breakthroughs. Cherish this time because it's temporary and allow yourself to handle what you can as you can.

GLOSSARY

ADLs (Activities of Daily Living): Basic essential tasks that need to be fulfilled to maintain one's basic needs, such as eating, bathing, toileting, dressing, grooming, and transferring.

Advance Directive (AD): Document in which the dementia patient explains their wishes and directs how their medical treatment should function. The AD is written and signed while the person is still in possession of their mental faculties.

Agnosia: When the dementia patient fails to recognize people and things through the use of their five senses.

Alzheimer's Disease: The most common cause of dementia in the US, Alzheimer's is a progressive disease that affects memory, thinking, and behavior. Alzheimer's development is often slow, and with time can make common daily tasks impossible.

Anomia: A difficulty to remember how objects are called, which can evolve to mixing the names of things with similar features.

Anosognosia: When one is incapable of understanding that they are physically or neurological impaired.

Apathy: Absence of interest, enthusiasm, or concern.

Appropriate care: The type of care that's selected among all existing types as the one that can offer the most benefit to a specific dementia patient.

Apraxia: Becoming unable to perform complex, learned, familiar, and purposeful movements. People with apraxia may also forget the order of common objects, causing behaviors such as putting a tie under a shirt.

Assessment: The ongoing process of evaluating the person's capacity of living independently and how much help they require.

Automatic thinking scripts: The capacity of completing routine tasks automatically. We all fulfill these scripts without rationalizing each step, which is acquired by repetition. This ability isn't lost with dementia, and the person can fulfill these tasks as long as they're in the same setting and there's no interruption.

Behavioral and Psychological Symptoms of Dementia (BPSD): Disruptive actions from the dementia patient caused by an unmet need. They can manifest as aggressions, compulsions, paranoia, and other unwanted behaviors.

Care Plan: An outline detailing the care goals for people with dementia, by analyzing their physical and psychosocial strengths and weaknesses. This document needs to be developed together with the patients, their families, and any medical specialist that's taking care of the case.

Challenging Behavior: Harsh behavior from the dementia patient, which has the potential of harm or disturb those around them, especially their family and caregivers. This behavior may be born from the frustration of the dementia patient to communicate with those around them.

Creutzfeldt Jacob Disease (CJD): An extremely rare condition caused by the alteration of body proteins by rogue prions, which affects the brain and nervous system.

Cognition: The ensemble of the perceptions that allow us to rationalize and understand ourselves and the world around us.

Cueing: Verbal or visual hints that communicate with the person of dementia so they can start or complete a task. It could be a sentence that makes them turn out the TV and go to bed, or having their outfit laid down in front of them as a cue that they should get dressed.

Delusion: A fixation that an illogical and false situation is true. Delusions often occur when the person mixes and distorts things that actually happen.

Dementia: A term that encompasses several symptoms connected with the loss of memory and cognition, which can be caused by a disease such Alzheimer's, or by a physical injury to the brain.

Depression: An unnatural feeling of sadness and hopelessness that's different from normal daily changes of mood. Depression happens with no apparent reason, though it can be increased by stress, abuse, drug and alcohol abuse, or the loss of a loved one.

Dysarthria: Difficulty to form words and sentences caused by the weakening of the speech muscles.

Dysphasia: Difficulty in understanding what others say.

Dysphagia: Difficulty in swallowing.

Electroencephalography (EEG): Medical test that measures electrical activity in the brain.

Experiential self: The part of our consciousness that is aware of the world around us, and absorbs its stimuli through our five physical senses.

Fight-or-flight response: An acute state of mind that happens when we're in a scary situation. The brain will then release hormones that will allow you to confront that situation or run away until you find a safe place.

Frontal Lobe: The part of the brain behind the forehead that controls emotions, personality, and cognition.

Frontotemporal dementia: A rare type of dementia that affects the frontal lobe of people between their thirties and sixties, affecting their social behavior and capacity of speech. People with frontotemporal dementia are often agitated and incur obsessive and repetitive behavior, but their memory isn't affected during the first stages of the disease.

Gait: An individual's personal walking pattern, which can be affected by dementia to the point of making the person disabled.

Habilitative care: A type of care in which the patient's abilities and disabilities are taken into account, and the environment around is changed in accordance. This helps the patient to retain some autonomy, and be able to fulfill their daily tasks with dignity.

Hallucination: A visual, auditory, or olfactory perception of something that's not there. Alzheimer's patients are prone to have hallucinations.

HIPAA: A document through which the dementia patients consent a third party to use or disclose their protected health information

Hippocampus: Part of the brain that generates short-term memory and emotions.

History: Medical and psycho-social history serve to detail previous treatments and incidents that the person has gone through, as to facilitate further treatment.

Huntington's Disease: A rare disease that causes involuntary movements and can develop into dementia. Huntington's disease appears in people between ages 30–45 years, and limits their life expectancy in fifteen more years.

Incontinence: Incapacity of controlling bladder and bowel functions. This is a common symptom in Alzheimer's patients, and can be treated in its early stages, though the use of geriatric diaper may become necessary.

Instrumental Activities of Daily Living (IADLs): Home management activities that improve people's lives in a community, though they are not as crucial as the ADLs. It includes housekeeping, financial management, preparing meals, getting around in a vehicle or public transportation, managing medicines, etc.

Intuitive thought processes: Thought process that happens in the right side of the brain, and which happens spontaneously and instantaneously, without requiring effort. Through the intuitive process, we get feelings, impressions, and instinctive responses, even if those contradict our rational feelings. Intuitive thought processes are fueled by our past experiences, and they allow us to enjoy art and beauty.

Korsakoff's Syndrome: Degenerative brain disease caused by alcohol abuse, which can affect short-term memory and make it hard to learn new skills.

Level of Care: Divided into mild (or "early"), moderate (or "middle"), and severe (or "late") this term reflects the amount of care that a person needs at a given point of their dementia treatment. The level of care is usually low at the moment of the diagnosis, but symptoms get worse as the disease progresses, and it's important to know when and how to get help.

Lewy Body Dementia: The second most common type of dementia, Lewy Body is caused by protein deposits in the nervous system, which affects memory, thinking, and movements. In late stages, the person suffers from visual hallucinations and symptoms associated with Parkinson's disease, such as tremors, rigid muscles, trouble walking, and slow movements.

Living Will: A document written and signed by a dementia patient after the diagnosis, but while they're still in control of their cognitive abilities. Through the living will, the dementia patient states their medical wishes and makes provisions for legal matters that may arise when they are not fully conscious anymore.

Long Term Memory: Memory that can be stored indefinitely, holding an unlimited amount of information.

Mild Cognitive Impairment (MCI): A cognitive problem that can be perceived, but is not strong enough to have a harmful impact on a person's life.

Mindfulness: The basic human ability of being conscious of the world around, being present, and perceiving things around you. It can be achieved through meditation and mental exercises.

Mindlessness: The opposite of mindfulness—being unaware of what you're doing, making unconscious decisions because your mind is wandering.

Magnetic Resonance Imaging (MRI): Radiology technique that uses body magnetism and computers to get images from inside the body, including the brain, which is valuable in dementia diagnosis and prognosis.

Muscle memory: The ability of remembering and repeating a task by following a pattern of movements without being conscious of it. Muscle memory is an enemy of mindfulness, and it can be broken by an unexpected situation that arises while you perform your task.

Neurodegenerative: Diseases that affect the structure and functioning of the brain tissue. Neurodegenerative diseases are more common in the elderly, but can show up in younger people.

Neurology: Medicine field that deals with the nervous system.

Occipital Lobe: Part of the brain that controls sight and the capacity of recognizing things. Located at the lower rear of the bran.

Paranoia: An acute feeling of suspicion without rational reasoning behind it.

Parietal Lobes: Part of the brain responsible for touch, pressure, pain, temperature, and taste. Located at the upper rear of the brain.

Parkinson's Disease: Neurological disorder that interferes with muscle, affecting gait and facial features, as well as causing tremors. Parkinson usually occurs during the early sixties, and moves slowly and progressively, and can cause symptoms of dementia.

Pathology: Field of medicine that studies diseases, establishing its causes, symptoms, and effects, by examining their impacts on the body.

Perception: Recognizing external stimuli through the five senses and interpreting them through an unconscious memory association.

Person-Centered Care: A type of dementia care that's based on each person's unique traits. The caregiver will take the person's life story and personality into account when planning and executing their activities, instead of following a pre-made formula.

Pick's Disease: Neurodegenerative disease that's a type of frontotemporal dementia, affecting the frontal and temporal lobes of the brain. It usually hits people between their 40' and 65's, first affecting the speech, then memory, and personality.

Plaques & Tangles: Interferences between the transmission of neurons, caused by Alzheimer's disease, preventing the neural system to exchange signals to each other. Plaques and tangles can only be identified during an autopsy.

Psychosocial: The psychological and social aspects related to a person's behavior.

Psychotropic Drugs: Drugs that have an effect on the brain, influencing a person's mental health. They can be antidepressant, anxiolytics, tranquilizers, and other drugs that have an effect on the patient's emotions and behavior.

Rational Thought Processes: These processes happen on the left side of the brain, and are responsible for methodical choices, interpretations, prioritizing actions and information, and following steps to achieve a goal. This kind of thought requires effort, and can tell us if we are having proper behavior during a situation, and how to act from there.

Remembering-self: A narrative used to make sense of our own history by reinterpreting nostalgic elements of ourselves to create a familiarity of our current surroundings.

Strength-based care: Treatment based on encouraging the use of the set of skills that a person continues to have while their dementia progresses. Knowing what these skills are helps caregivers to develop activities for that person, which benefits their experience.

Sundowning Syndrome: Sensation of disorientation and irritability that some people with dementia have when the sun goes down at the end of the day. Its causes are not clear, but could have to do with the change in the environment or the feeling of tiredness.

Temporal Lobes: Part of the brain responsible for audition, also connected with memory, language, emotion, interpretation, and learning. Located above the ears.

Vascular Dementia: Type of dementia caused by several small strokes, which are often not perceived, but can have an impact in the brain.

Wandering: Moving around aimlessly without goal or direction, which can bring a person of dementia to exhaustion or take them to a place where their security is at risk. It's possible to wander safely if there's an appropriate space for that, such as a garden or a backyard.

Ward of Court: A person appointed by the court to manage the affairs of a dementia patient who has been declared legally incapable of doing that themselves.

REFERENCES

Aarp, A. G. (n.d.). *Time management for the caregiver.* AARP. https://www.aarp.org/home-family/caregiving/info-2016/time-management-for-caregiver.html

About epilepsy | CDC. (n.d.). https://www.cdc.gov/epilepsy/about/

Activities for dementia. (2021, December 8). nhs.uk. https://www.nhs.uk/conditions/dementia/activities/

Alzheimer's and dementia: Tips for better communication. (2021, March 12). Mayo Clinic. https://www.mayoclinic.org/healthy-lifestyle/caregivers/in-depth/alzheimers/art-20047540

Alzheimer's Disease: common medical problems. (n.d.). National Institute on Aging. https://www.nia.nih.gov/health/alzheimers-disease-common-medical-problems

Alzheimer's disease facts and figures. (n.d.). Alzheimer's Association. https://www.alz.org/alzheimers-dementia/facts-figures

Alzheimer's: Managing sleep problems. (2021, December 3). Mayo Clinic. https://www.mayoclinic.org/healthy-lifestyle/caregivers/in-depth/alzheimers/art-20047832

Bathrooms - Dementia-friendly environments - SCIE. (2020, October). Social Care Institute for Excellence. https://www.scie.org.uk/dementia/supporting-people-with-dementia/dementia-friendly-environments/toilets-and-bathrooms.asp

Behavior & personality Changes. (n.d.). Memory and Aging Center. https://memory.ucsf.edu/caregiving-support/behavior-personality-changes

The benefits of socialization for people with dementia | The Arbors - The Ivy. (2023, June 21). *The* Arbors & The Ivy Assisted Living. https://arborsassistedliving.com/the-benefits-of-socialization-for-people-with-dementia

Birt, C. (2021, September 28). *Bathroom safety for Alzheimer's & dementia.* Carewell. https://www.carewell.com/resources/blog/bathroom-safety-alzheimers-dementia

Blane, P. (2023, June 14). *When should dementia patients stop living alone?* Care Business Associate Training. https://cbassociatetraining.co.uk/when-should-dementia-patients-stop-living-alone

Brady, K. (2020, September 9). *10 Ways to increase intimacy in your relationship - Keir Brady Counseling Services.* Keir Brady Counseling Services. https://keirbradycounseling.com/10-ways-to-increase-intimacy/

Bridges to Recovery. (2020). 6 ways to support someone with major depression.

Bridges to Recovery. https://www.bridgestorecovery.com/blog/6-ways-support-someone-major-depression

Brodaty, H., & Donkin, M. (2009). Family caregivers of people with dementia. *Dialogues in Clinical Neuroscience, 11*(2), 217–228. https://doi.org/10.31887/dcns.2009.11.2/hbrodaty

Cafasso, J. (2023, February 23). *12 tips for a speedy flu recovery.* Healthline. https://www.healthline.com/health/influenza/tips-for-speedy-flu-recovery

Caregiver statistics: Demographics - family caregiver alliance. (2022, December 2). Family Caregiver Alliance. https://www.caregiver.org/resource/caregiver-statistics-demographics/

Communicating with someone with dementia. (2023, February 24). nhs.uk. https://www.nhs.uk/conditions/dementia/communication-and-dementia/

Communication and Alzheimer's. (n.d.). Alzheimer's Disease and Dementia. https://www.alz.org/help-support/caregiving/daily-care/communications

Coxwell, K. (2022). How to deal with dementia or Alzheimer's: 5 retirement financial planning steps. *NewRetirement.* https://www.newretirement.com/retirement/how-to-deal-with-dementia-or-alzheimers-5-retirement-financial-planning-steps/

The dangers of dehydration for seniors. (n.d.). Integris Health. https://integrisok.com/resources/on-your-health/2019/september/the-dangers-of-dehydration-for-seniors

De Jonghe-Rouleau, A. P., Pot, A. M., & De Jonghe, J. F. M. (2005). Self-injurious Behaviour in nursing home residents with dementia. *International Journal of Geriatric Psychiatry, 20*(7), 651–657. https://doi.org/10.1002/gps.1337

Dementia. (2023, March 15). www.who.int. https://www.who.int/news-room/fact-sheets/detail/dementia

Dementia - activities and exercise. (n.d.). Better Health Channel. https://www.betterhealth.vic.gov.au/health/conditionsandtreatments/dementia-activities-and-exercise

Dementia - behavior changes. (n.d.). Better Health Channel. https://www.betterhealth.vic.gov.au/health/conditionsandtreatments/dementia-behaviour-changes

Dementia - hygiene. (n.d.). Better Health Channel. https://www.betterhealth.vic.gov.au/health/conditionsandtreatments/dementia-hygiene

Dementia - Symptoms and causes - Mayo Clinic. (2023, June 22). Mayo Clinic. https://www.mayoclinic.org/diseases-conditions/dementia/symptoms-causes/syc-20352013

Dementia: 7 stages. (n.d.). Compassion & Choices. https://www.compassionandchoices.org/resource/dementia-7-stages

Dementia nurse interview questions and answers. (n.d.). https://fixedcareer.com/dementia-nurse-interview-questions/

Dementia planning is an important part of estate planning. (2022, August 18).

Moneyweb. https://www.moneyweb.co.za/financial-advisor-views/dementia-planning-is-an-important-part-of-estate-planning/

Dementia Terminology. (2023, May 30). The Good Care Group. https://www.thegoodcaregroup.com/live-in-care/dementia-care/dementia-terminology/

DementiaCareCentral.com (2023, January 26). *Stages of Alzheimer's & dementia: Durations & scales used to measure progression (GDS, FAST & CDR).* www.dementiacarecentral.com. https://www.dementiacarecentral.com/aboutdementia/facts/stages

Dementia-friendly communities. (n.d.). Alzheimer's Society. https://www.alzheimers.org.uk/get-involved/dementia-friendly-communities/

Dementia-friendly faith groups. (n.d.). Alzheimer's Society. https://www.alzheimers.org.uk/get-involved/dementia-friendly-communities/faith-groups

Dementia Terminology. (n.d.). The Good Care Group. https://www.thegoodcaregroup.com/live-in-care/dementia-care/dementia-terminology/

Derrick. (2022, March 25). Alzheimer's disease kitchen safety - checklist. *Elder Guru.* https://www.elderguru.com/alzheimers-disease-kitchen-safety-checklist

Dizziness and fainting with dementia - Lifted. (2023, March 10). Lifted. https://www.liftedcare.com/news/dizziness-and-fainting-with-dementia/

Eating and nutritional challenges in patients with Alzheimer's disease: Tips for caregivers. (n.d.). Cleveland Clinic. https://my.clevelandclinic.org/health/articles/9597-eating-and-nutritional-challenges-in-patients-with-alzheimers-disease-tips-for-caregivers

Efetherston. (2021). *UNderstanding behavioral changes in dementia.* Lewy Body Dementia Association. https://www.lbda.org/understanding-behavioral-changes-in-dementia/

8 helpful tips for time management - Caregiver Solutions Magazine. (2022, August 25). Caregiver Solutions Magazine. https://www.caregiversolutions.ca/caregiving/8-helpful-tips-for-time-management

11 ways to get someone with dementia to take medication. (2023, June 5). DailyCaring. https://dailycaring.com/11-ways-to-get-someone-with-dementia-to-take-medication/

Falls and dementia. (n.d.). NHS Inform. https://www.nhsinform.scot/healthy-living/preventing-falls/falls-and-dementia

Feeding and nutrition (for dementia) - Family Caregiver Alliance. (2021, August 19). Family Caregiver Alliance. https://www.caregiver.org/resource/feeding-and-nutrition-dementia

50 activities. (n.d.). Alzheimer's Disease and Dementia. https://www.alz.org/help-support/resources/kids-teens/50-activities

Food and eating. (n.d.). Alzheimer's Disease and Dementia. https://www.alz.org/help-support/caregiving/daily-care/food-eating

Functional assessment staging tool for dementia | Resources. (2023, February 14). Compassus. https://www.compassus.com/healthcare-professionals/determining-eligibility/functional-assessment-staging-tool-fast-scale-for-dementia/

Get involved with your local chapter. (n.d.). Alzheimer's Disease and Dementia. https://www.alz.org/local_resources/find_your_local_chapter

Glen Campbell's daughter on the hardships of Alzheimer's. (2015, March 10). [Video]. NBC News. https://www.nbcnews.com/health/aging/glen-campbell-family-feud-dementia-divides-many-clans-n320416

Going to the hospital: Tips for dementia caregivers. (n.d.). National Institute on Aging. https://www.nia.nih.gov/health/going-hospital-tips-dementia-caregivers

Grief and loss as Alzheimer's progresses. (n.d.). Alzheimer's Disease and Dementia. https://www.alz.org/help-support/caregiving/caregiver-health/grief-loss-as-alzheimers-progresses

Hales, M. (2020, February 18). *HIPAA authorization required.* The HIPAA E-TOOL®. https://thehipaaetool.com/hipaa-authorization-required/

Hanlon Niemann & Wright, P.C. (2022, March 26). *Glossary of terms for alzheimer's & dementia | Hanlon Niemann & Wright.* Hanlon Niemann & Wright Law Firm | New Jersey Attorneys. https://www.hnwlaw.com/elder-law/dementia-alzheimers-law/glossary-of-terms-for-alzheimers-dementia/

Heerema, E. H. (2022, April 23). *DOor alarms for wandering in Alzheimer's and dementia.* Verywell Health. https://www.verywellhealth.com/safety-in-dementia-door-alarms-98172

Hitt, R. (2023, May 15). *Importance of routine for dementia | Where you live matters.* ASHA. https://www.whereyoulivematters.org/importance-of-routines-for-dementia

Hobson, G. (2023). *Dealing with dementia behaviors: Tips for understanding and coping.* www.aplaceformom.com. https://www.aplaceformom.com/caregiver-resources/articles/dementia-behaviors

Home safety checklist for Alzheimer's disease. (n.d.). National Institute on Aging. https://www.nia.nih.gov/health/home-safety-checklist-alzheimers-disease

How are dementia, Alzheimer's disease and seizures linked? | Epilepsy blog. (n.d.). https://www.epsyhealth.com/seizure-epilepsy-blog/how-are-dementia-alzheimers-disease-and-seizures-linked

How to communicate with a person with dementia. (2021, December 20). Alzheimer's Society. https://www.alzheimers.org.uk/about-dementia/symptoms-and-diagnosis/symptoms/how-to-communicate-dementia

How to talk to the doctor about your elderly parent or spouse. (n.d.). © 2007-2023 AgingCare All Rights Reserved. https://www.agingcare.com/articles/doctor-visits-with-elderly-parent-149071.htm

In-home Alzheimer's care & dementia care service | Nurse next door. (n.d.). Nurse Next Door Senior Care Services. https://www.nursenextdoor.com/our-services/alzheimers-dementia-care/

In-home care. (n.d.). Alzheimer's Disease and Dementia. https://www.alz.org/help-support/caregiving/care-options/in-home-care

Jozefiak, M. (2023, April 14). *7 Best remote support groups for caregivers of people with dementia.* Caregiver Support and Resources. https://www.careforth.com/blog/7-best-remote-support-groups-for-caregivers-of-people-with-dementia

Kaput, K. (2023, June 12). *Self-Care tips for caregivers: Your health matters, too.* Cleveland Clinic. https://health.clevelandclinic.org/self-care-for-caregivers/

Kazanowski, K. A. (2021, September 27). *Ending the Family Feud.* Caregiver.com. https://caregiver.com/articles/ending-family-feud/

Keeping safe: fire, cooking and kitchens. (n.d.). Alzheimer's Society. https://www.alzheimers.org.uk/get-support/staying-independent/fire-risk-cooking-kitchens

Leaves, A. (2014, May 15). *5 simple ways to help someone with dementia in the short and Long term - Autumn Leaves.* Autumn Leaves. https://autumnleaves.com/5-simple-ways-help-someone-dementia-short-long-term/

Legal documents. (n.d.). Alzheimer's Disease and Dementia. https://www.alz.org/help-support/caregiving/financial-legal-planning/legal-documents

Lesser known symptoms of dementia | Alzheimer Scotland. (2022, May 27). Alzheimer Scotland. https://www.alzscot.org/lesser-known-symptoms-of-dementia

Lewy body dementia - Symptoms and causes - Mayo Clinic. (2023, June 2). Mayo Clinic. https://www.mayoclinic.org/diseases-conditions/lewy-body-dementia/symptoms-causes/syc-20352025

Lobes of the brain. (2018, July 17). Queensland Brain Institute - University of Queensland. https://qbi.uq.edu.au/brain/brain-anatomy/lobes-brain

Managing family conflicts when a parent is diagnosed with dementia. (2020). Livewell Estates | Dementia and Alzheimer's Care. https://livewell.care/managing-family-conflicts-when-a-parent-is-diagnosed-with-dementia

Marquand, B. (2023, March 20). *Long-term care insurance explained.* NerdWallet. https://www.nerdwallet.com/article/insurance/long-term-care-insurance

Memory, forgetfulness, and aging: What's normal and what's not? (n.d.). National Institute on Aging. https://www.nia.nih.gov/health/memory-forgetfulness-and-aging-whats-normal-and-whats-not

Mental, physical and speech abilities in later stages of dementia. (2022, June 29). Alzheimer's Society. https://www.alzheimers.org.uk/about-dementia/symptoms-and-diagnosis/how-dementia-progresses/mental-and-physical-activities

Morrisette, S. (2023). *12 top tips: Effective time management for caregivers.* Smartcare Software. https://smartcaresoftware.com/news/12-top-tips-effective-time-management-for-caregivers/

Nadine, N. (2023, January 24). *Questions to ask your doctor after an elderly person falls.* Winfar Mobility Products & Home Care Aids. https://winfar.co.za/questions-to-ask-your-doctor-after-an-elderly-person-falls/

Nao. (2023). *Occipital lobe dementia: Symptoms, causes, and treatment* | Nao Medical. Nao Medical. https://naomedical.com/blog/occipital-lobe-dementia-symptoms-causes-treatment-nao-medical/

New drug for Alzheimer's slows down cognitive decline in key trial. (2022, September 28). [Video]. NBC News. https://www.nbcnews.com/health/aging/alzheimers-drug-slowed-progression-disease-phase-3-trial-rcna49689

9 kitchen safety tips to keep your senior safe and comfortable. (2021, August 20). https://www.completecareatlanta.com/9-kitchen-safety-tips-to-keep-your-senior-safe-and-comfortable

Ninkatec. (2023, April 14). *Caring for your dementia loved one: Tips from professional nurses* | Ninkatec. Ninkatec. https://ninkatec.com/dementia-home-care-tips-from-professional-nurses/

Oral health for older adults: quick tips - MyHealthFinder | Health.gov. (2019, June 1). https://health.gov/myhealthfinder/doctor-visits/regular-checkups/oral-health-older-adults-quick-tips

Pain in advanced dementia - SCIE. (n.d.). https://www.scie.org.uk/dementia/advanced-dementia-and-end-of-life-care/end-of-life-care/pain.asp

Physical exercise and dementia | Dementia care tips. (n.d.). Homewatch CareGivers. https://www.homewatchcaregivers.com/dementia/living-with-dementia/physical-exercise/

The psychological and emotional impact of dementia. (2022, June 27). Alzheimer's Society. https://www.alzheimers.org.uk/get-support/help-dementia-care/understanding-supporting-person-dementia-psychological-emotional-impact

Planning ahead for legal matters. (n.d.). Alzheimer's Disease and Dementia. https://www.alz.org/help-support/caregiving/financial-legal-planning/planning-ahead-for-legal-matters

Primary care for your loved one with Alzheimer's. (2018, August 21). WebMD. https://www.webmd.com/alzheimers/alzheimers-medical-office-visits

Quotes for dementia caregivers in need of inspiration | ActivePro Nursing & Homecare Inc. | Niagara. (2018, July 10). https://www.nursehomecare.ca/site/blog/2018/07/10/homecare-services-inspirational-quotes-for-dementia-caregivers

Rasmussen, J., & Langerman, H. (2019). Alzheimer's Disease – Why We Need Early Diagnosis. *Degenerative Neurological and Neuromuscular Disease, Volume 9*, 123–130.

Rehman, A. (2022, July 25). *Neuroanatomy, occipital lobe.* National Laboratory of Medicine. https://www.ncbi.nlm.nih.gov/books/NBK544320

Resolving family conflicts. (n.d.). Alzheimer's Disease and Dementia. https://www.alz.org/help-support/resources/resolving-family-conflicts

Self-Care for caregivers. (2022, June 24). ucsfhealth.org. https://www.ucsfhealth.org/education/self-care-for-caregivers

Sight and hearing loss with dementia. (n.d.). Alzheimer's Society. https://www.alzheimers.org.uk/about-dementia/symptoms-and-diagnosis/sight-hearing-loss

6 easy ways to make a dementia-safe kitchen - Lifted. (2021, May 4). Lifted. https://www.liftedcare.com/news/6-easy-ways-to-make-a-dementia-safe-kitchen

6 Self-care tips for caregivers. (n.d.). https://www.betterup.com/blog/self-care-for-caregivers

The 6 r's of managing difficult behavior (From the 36-hour day). (2010, January 6). Brain Support Network. https://www.brainsupportnetwork.org/the-6-rs-of-managing-difficult-behavior-from-the-36-hour-day

Skin care tips for those with Alzheimer's disease. (2015, April 23). Alzheimer's, Education, Caregivers. https://www.alzu.org/blog/2015/04/23/skin-care-tips-for-those-with-alzheimer

Sleep issues and sundowning. (n.d.). Alzheimer's Disease and Dementia. https://www.alz.org/help-support/caregiving/stages-behaviors/sleep-issues-sundowning

Smith, S. (2018, October 4). *5-4-3-2-1 coping technique for anxiety.* https://www.urmc.rochester.edu/behavioral-health-partners/bhp-blog/april-2018/5-4-3-2-1-coping-technique-for-anxiety.aspx

Sollitto, M. (n.d.). *3 Legal documents caregivers need to manage a senior's health care.* AgingCare. https://www.agingcare.com/articles/legal-documents-to-make-healthcare-decisions-for-your-parent-146623.htm

Spriggs, B. B. (2017, August 4). *Alzheimer's disease doctors.* Healthline. https://www.healthline.com/health/alzheimers-disease-doctors

Staff, C. (2022). *9 caregiver support groups that help caregivers in need.* Caring-Bridge. https://www.caringbridge.org/resources/caregiver-support-groups/

Starkman, E. (2022, August 25). *Socializing and activities for loved ones with Alzheimer's.* WebMD. https://www.webmd.com/alzheimers/socializing-activities-alzheimers

Staying physically active with Alzheimer's. (n.d.). National Institute on Aging. https://www.nia.nih.gov/health/staying-physically-active-alzheimers

Stuart, A. (2012, July 5). *Brain exercises and dementia.* WebMD. https://www.webmd.com/alzheimers/guide/preventing-dementia-brain-exercises

Support groups. (n.d.). Alzheimer's Disease and Dementia. https://www.alz.org/help-support/community/support-groups

Taking care of you: Self-care for family caregivers - Family Caregiver Alliance. (2023, January 11). Family Caregiver Alliance. https://www.caregiver.org/resource/taking-care-you-self-care-family-caregivers/

Tee-Melegrito, R. A. (2022, August 23). *Tips for talking to someone with dementia.*

https://www.medicalnewstoday.com/articles/how-to-talk-to-someone-with-dementia

The 10 benefits of early diagnosis. (n.d.). Alzheimer Society of Canada. https://alzheimer.ca/en/about-dementia/do-i-have-dementia/how-get-tested-dementia/10-benefits-early-diagnosis

30 physician interview questions and answers for 2023. (2023, March 31). https://bemoacademicconsulting.com/blog/physician-interview-questions

Tips for spending quality time with your child. (n.d.). NAEYC. https://www.naeyc.org/our-work/families/spending-quality-time-with-your-child

Understanding how your relationship may change. (n.d.). Alzheimer Society of Canada. https://alzheimer.ca/en/help-support/i-have-friend-or-family-member-who-lives-dementia/understanding-how-your-relationship

Van Hook, M. (2022, March 26). *Making a dementia care plan: 10 questions to ask your doctor.* The Arbor Company. https://www.arborcompany.com/blog/making-dementia-care-plan-10-questions-to-ask

VAscular dementia: Causes, symptoms, and treatments. (n.d.). National Institute on Aging. https://www.nia.nih.gov/health/vascular-dementia

Wang, J. J., Wang, C. J., Chang, L. H., & Yang, Y. Y. (2022). Want model: The need-centered care and management model for behavioral and psychological symptoms dementia. *Journal of Clinical Epigenetics, 7*(9.004).

Waters, S. (2022, September 7). *6 self-care tips for caregivers.* Better Up. https://www.betterup.com/blog/self-care-for-caregivers

Wetherell, J. L., & Jeste, D. V. (2003). Diagnostic decision tree in dementia. Dialogues in Clinical Neuroscience, 5(1), 44–47. https://doi.org/10.31887/dcns.2003.5.1/jloebachwetherell

What are frontotemporal disorders? Causes, symptoms, and treatment. (n.d.). National Institute on Aging. https://www.nia.nih.gov/health/what-are-frontotemporal-disorders

What are the seven stages of dementia? | IP Homecare. (2021, October 12). IP Homecare. https://www.ip-live-in-care.co.uk/7-stages-dementia/

What is a geriatric care manager? (n.d.). National Institute on Aging. https://www.nia.nih.gov/health/what-geriatric-care-manager

What is a living trust? (2022, September 16). https://www.investopedia.com/terms/l/living-trust.asp

What is Alzheimer's? (n.d.). Alzheimer's Disease and Dementia. https://www.alz.org/alzheimers-dementia/what-is-alzheimers

What is dementia? (n.d.). Alzheimer's Disease and Dementia. https://www.alz.org/alzheimers-dementia/what-is-dementia

What is dementia? | CDC. (n.d.). https://www.cdc.gov/aging/dementia/index.html

What is dementia? Symptoms, types, and diagnosis. (n.d.). National Institute on Aging. https://www.nia.nih.gov/health/what-is-dementia

What Is Lewy Body dementia? Causes, symptoms, and treatments. (n.d.). National

Institute on Aging. https://www.nia.nih.gov/health/what-lewy-body-dementia-causes-symptoms-and-treatments

What is mixed dementia? (n.d.). Alzheimer's Society. https://www.alzheimers.org.uk/blog/what-is-mixed-dementia

What not to say to somebody with dementia. (n.d.). Alzheimer's Society. https://www.alzheimers.org.uk/blog/language-dementia-what-not-to-say

White, S. (2020). 9 great time management tips for caregivers. *Caregiver Warrior.* https://www.caregiverwarrior.com/9-great-time-management-tips-for-caregivers/

Whitley, M. (2023). How to talk to someone with dementia: 10 expert Alzheimer's communication Strategies. *www.aplaceformom.com.* https://www.aplaceformom.com/caregiver-resources/articles/dementia-communication

Why early diagnosis is important - Dementia - SCIE. (n.d.). https://www.scie.org.uk/dementia/symptoms/diagnosis/early-diagnosis.asp

Women as carers: gender considerations and stigma in dementia care. (n.d.). Alzheimer's Disease National. https://www.alzint.org/news-events/news/women-as-carers-gender-considerations-and-stigma-in-dementia-care/

Yang, X., Vedel, I., & Khanassov, V. (2021). The Cultural Diversity of Dementia Patients and Caregivers in Primary Care Case Management: a Pilot Mixed Methods Study. *Canadian Geriatrics Journal, 24*(3), 184–194. https://doi.org/10.5770/cgj.24.490

Made in the USA
Las Vegas, NV
19 November 2023

81160126R00085